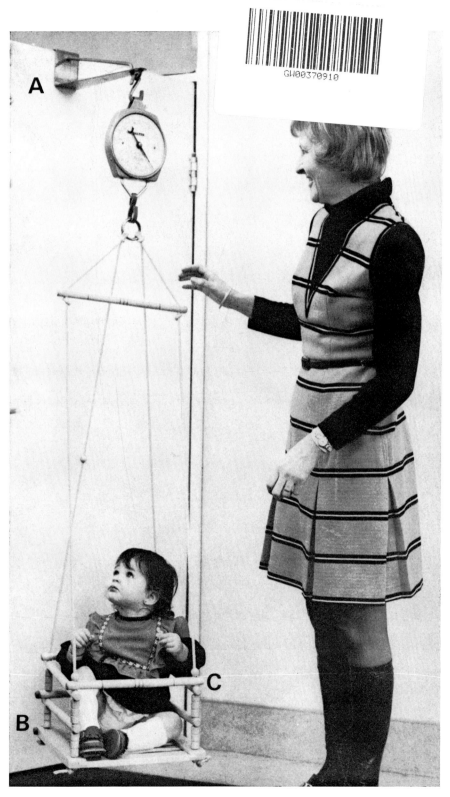

Frontispiece 1   Measurement of weight (see page 116)

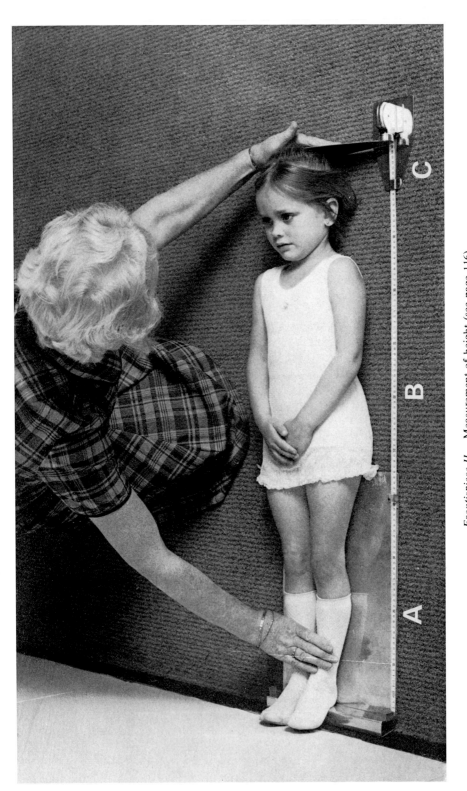

Frontispiece II Measurement of height (see page 116)

Department of Health and Social Security

Report on Health and Social Subjects
10

A NUTRITION SURVEY OF PRE-SCHOOL CHILDREN, 1967-68

Report by the Committee on Medical Aspects of Food Policy

London
Her Majesty's Stationery Office

ISBN 0 11 320603 8

Personnel involved in the Survey

The survey was commissioned by the Committee on Medical Aspects of Food Policy. It was planned and carried out by the following members of the staffs of the British Market Research Bureau, the Department of Health and Social Security (then the Ministry of Health), the Scottish Home and Health Department, the Social Survey Division of the Office of Population Censuses and Surveys (then the Government Social Survey) and the Welsh Office Health and Social Work Department (then the Welsh Board of Health) with advice from some observers:

Dr. W. T. C. Berry, CBE   Department of Health and Social Security
London

Mrs. M. E. Cadman   Department of Health and Social Security
London

Mrs. K. Daniels   Department of Health and Social Security
London

Dr. S. J. Darke   Department of Health and Social Security
London

Mrs. M. M. Disselduff   Department of Health and Social Security
London

Mr. F. J. Downer   Department of Health and Social Security
London

Dr. J. V. G. A. Durnin   Institute of Physiology
University of Glasgow

Mrs. J. M. Firth   Department of Health and Social Security
London

Mr. J. E. Fothergill   British Market Research Bureau
London

Dr. M. M. Gray (d. 1973)   Welsh Board of Health
Cardiff

Miss D. F. Hollingsworth   Ministry of Agriculture, Fisheries and Food
London

(Now Director of the British Nutrition Foundation)

Miss P. M. Hurley

Department of Health and Social Security
London

Mrs. S. Keith

Department of Health and Social Security
London

Mr. W. F. F. Kemsley

Social Survey Division of the Office of
Population Censuses and Surveys
London

Miss J. Marr

Social Medicine Research Unit,
London School of Hygiene and Tropical
Medicine

Dr. M. E. Mitchell
(retired, 1971)

Scottish Home and Health Department
Edinburgh

Dr. E. La C. Murphy

Department of Health and Social Security
London

Miss J. Robertson

Ministry of Agriculture, Fisheries and Food
London

Mr. J. Rodgers

Department of Health and Social Security
London

Preface

In the early 1960s the Committee on Medical Aspects of Food Policy was con-concerned about the nutritional status of those members of the population who might be considered, for one reason or another, to be at risk of sub-optimal nutrition. A series of nutrition surveys was therefore planned. At the time the methodology both of drawing a random sample and of carrying out such a study in the pre-school years was thought to warrant a pilot study. This was made in 1963, but the analysis of the results and the planning of nutrition surveys of other age groups in the light of what was learned about methodology took a long time and the main survey of pre-school children commissioned by the Committee on Medical Aspects of Food Policy was not commenced until October 1967. The field work extended over one year and the random sample of 1 321 children aged six months to $4\frac{1}{2}$ years of age was representative of Great Britain as a whole.

This is the first study of its kind to be made in Britain on such young children. The only other comparable study was one in 1951 by Bransby and Fothergill, who surveyed a smaller number of children (461) in one month of the year only and in a smaller number of areas.

In the five years between the pilot study and the main study reported here much had been learned but, as in all such work, much more has been learned since, especially about the collection of anthropometric information. The Committee is fully aware that, given adequate staff, any such study could today be made with refinements in both the collection and analysis of information, but believes that this publication, late as it is, may be a valuable source of information and guidance for those who undertake future studies.

The results of the study produced no evidence that our pre-school children were underfed and this is true equally for the children of larger families in social classes IV and V and for the children of small families in social classes I and II. In fact the average daily intake of the energy-producing foods was higher in the former children although they were neither taller nor heavier on average than the children in social classes I and II; this may have been because their energy expenditure was greater.

The Committee is much indebted to all those who made the survey possible and brought it to a successful outcome.

G E GODBER
Chairman,
Committee on Medical Aspects of
Food Policy
September 1973

Acknowledgements

We are greatly indebted to all Medical Officers of Health who helped us with this survey for giving access to records, for assistance in providing the information necessary for selecting the sample and for providing facilities for the medical examinations; to the Chief Dental Officers and their staff for cooperation in the dental examinations, and to the field workers without whose help such a survey would not have been possible.

Contents

Index to Appendix A:
Detailed Tables and Diagrams

Tables

Index to Appendix B:
Forms used in the survey

1. Introduction

1.1 Early in the last decade, the Chief Medical Officer's Committee on Medical Aspects of Food Policy recommended a programme of nutrition surveys of those sections of the community which might be considered of special nutritional interest. One of these sections was pre-school children, and a pilot survey of 429 children between the ages of 9 months and 5 years was carried out between May and September 1963. Details of the methodology and results of this survey were published by the Ministry of Health (1968).

1.2 Much was learned from the pilot study both with regard to sampling technique and to the problems of a dietary study in the field. In the larger comprehensive survey reported here advantage was taken of what had been learned, although for purposes of comparison the techniques remained in essence the same. This survey extended over one year from October 1967 to September 1968.

1.3 The present report gives the nutritional findings on a sample of children representative of Great Britain as a whole; it includes details of methodology in order that the validity of the findings may be assessed.

2. The Sample

2.1 Structure

2.1.1 The aim was to obtain a nationally representative sample in each of 3 family size groups of children aged between 6 months and $4\frac{1}{2}$ years living with their families at home. Children living in institutions or in care, foster children, children attending nursery or other day schools and infants still being breast fed were excluded.

2.1.2 The family size groups by which the sample was stratified were families with one or two children, with three children and with four or more children under 15 years of age, including the sample child. The method of sampling made it unnecessary to stratify for sex and age. Only one child per household was included in the survey.

2.2 Method of obtaining the sample

2.2.1 The Social Survey Division of the Office of Population Censuses and Surveys (the then Government Social Survey) selected 39 areas in Great Britain each having a total population of the order of 100 000 which were regarded as corporately representative of the country as a whole. Four areas were in Scotland, 2 in Wales and 33 in England, including 5 in Greater London. The local authority areas in which they were situated were as follows:

England	Worcestershire	Newham
Cambridgeshire	Yorkshire (West Riding)	Richmond
Cheshire	Birmingham	Wandsworth
Derbyshire	Blackburn	
Dorset	Grimsby	*Wales*
Durham	Huddersfield	Carmarthenshire
Essex	Leeds	Glamorgan
Gloucestershire	Luton	
Hampshire	Manchester	*Scotland*
Kent	Northampton	Aberdeenshire
Lancashire (2 areas)	Nottingham	Fifeshire
Shropshire	Walsall	Midlothian
Staffordshire		Glasgow
Surrey	*Greater London*	
East Sussex	Barnet	
Warwickshire	Hackney	

2.2.2 The field work was organized so that all 39 areas would be covered in each quarter of the year by working on a monthly cycle of 13 areas, and in each month the same number of children (5 children in each of the three family size groups) would be included in each area. This gave a sample of 2 340 children, which was within the capacity of the available fieldwork resources and adequate from a statistical standpoint, after allowing for non-response on the scale experienced in the pilot survey.

2.2.3   In the 34 areas outside Greater London the sample was drawn quarterly by the British Market Research Bureau (employed by the then Government Social Survey to do the fieldwork) from the Welfare Milk application records held by local offices of the Ministry of Social Security, as it was then, covering the sample areas. (This method of sampling became impracticable in 1969, when these records ceased to be maintained on a local basis.) The record consisted of a card giving particulars of the mother and all the children in the family who were entitled to Welfare Milk, but not the information about any older children which was required for stratification purposes. Consequently, it was necessary to obtain this further information from the records of the local authorities in which the sample areas were situated.

2.2.4   To allow, therefore, for (a) deletion of those addresses in the sample areas which were situated outside the geographical area of the then Ministry of Social Security local offices; (b) deletion of any children outside the age limit of the survey, and (c) the estimated variation in family size (for which there was no reliable guide), a very much larger sample of records (over 27 000 in all) had to be extracted in the first place. A quarter of the cases still remaining after the deletion of (a) and (b) above had been made were sent to the local health authorities for addition of the information, when known, on siblings up to the age of 15. Adjustment was then made to maintain the correct probability of selection, and finally the number in each family size group for each month was reduced to 5 (para 2.2.2) by discarding at random. Despite the very large margin allowed for the various processes of adjustment and rejection, a few groups finished with less than 5 names, and this is the reason for the shortfall of 19 in the actual number selected (2 321).

2.2.5   In Greater London, because centralization of the Welfare Milk records had already taken place, it was not possible to use them for sampling. Instead, the sample was drawn by the then Ministry of Health staff in four quarterly batches from health visitors' records maintained by the local health authorities covering the five London sample areas. In most cases these records contained information on all children of school and pre-school age, enabling selection of the sample by family size to be made directly.

2.2.6   A disadvantage of this method of sampling was that it provided no information on the incidence of families of the three different sizes in the total population as defined for the survey. Consequently, it has not been possible to find a suitable basis for weighting the findings in respect of the three individual family size groups to produce adjusted data relating to all family sizes. In this report results are discussed either in terms of individual family size groups, particularly where the similarity (or the contrast) in their behaviour is of interest, or in terms of an unweighted combination of the family size group results.

3. Methodology of the Survey

3.1 Field work

3.1.1   The interviewing and supervision of the dietary recording was carried out by the British Market Research Bureau, after training in the methods established by the Ministry of Health. A month in each quarter of the year of the survey was spent in each area, and during this time the respondents were interviewed.

3.1.2   The interviewers obtained information about the child and the family. This included the composition of the household and the number of earners, the father's occupation and income, the age at which the mother completed her full-time education, whether Welfare Milk tokens were obtained, and any circumstances which might have affected the child's dietary pattern in the week of the survey. When consent was forthcoming, the child's height and weight and the heights of both parents were recorded. The questionnaire used to obtain this information is included in Appendix B1 (p 95).

3.1.3   The mothers (or guardians) of the children were asked to keep weighed records of all food and drink consumed by the children for a period of seven consecutive days (see specimen record book, Appendix B2, p 105). A system of cumulative weighing in ounces and sixths of ounces was used, and food scales, which had been specially calibrated in these units, were loaned to households. The weights of foods left over were also recorded and appropriate quantity units were used for the few items which were too small to weigh, so that the computer was able to calculate the total net intake of each food.

3.2 Food composition table

3.2.1   A revised and up-to-date version of the food composition table used in the pilot survey in 1963 (Ministry of Health, 1968, Appendix D) was prepared for this survey. As before, a weighted figure was used for those foods (e.g. potatoes) which were known to have a wide seasonal variation in nutrient content. Supplies of these foods come from many different countries and it was unrealistic to expect mothers to know the country of origin or age of the foods they purchased. Consequently, it was felt that any attempt to classify these foods on a seasonal basis would be no more, and perhaps less, precise than the application of one weighted figure.

3.2.2   Each of the 630 food codes had an attributed figure for energy value and for the nutrients listed in Tables A 7–10 (pp 41–44). In addition, where one of the principal animal protein contributing foods (milk, cheese, meat, eggs and fish) was a component of a mixed dish the percentage of this food was

4

defined. This allowed a total consumption of each of these foods (in whatever form consumed) to be calculated for each child.

3.2.3 Because of a possible relationship between sugar consumption and the prevalence of dental caries and of obesity, the food codes had an attributed figure not only for total carbohydrate expressed as monosaccharide but also for "added sugars". These are defined as any sugars consumed as such, or added during the cooking, preparation or manufacture of food as distinct from the naturally occurring carbohydrates of the basic foods. With a few exceptions, these sugars are added in the form of sucrose. The consumption of carbohydrate and of "added sugars" was listed for each child, total carbohydrate being expressed as monosaccharides and "added sugars" as disaccharides.

3.2.4 The food code list was divided into 26 food groups (Table A42, p 67), the groupings being based on similarity of composition of the individual foods. A simple list of nutrient intakes was thought to be of limited practical value unless the foods which provided these nutrients could be identified.

3.3 Medical and dental examinations

3.3.1 With permission from the mother or guardian, arrangements were made in appropriate cases for medical and for dental examinations. The forms used are reproduced in Appendices B3 and B4 (pp 112 and 114) and the results of the examinations are described in Appendices D and E (pp 117 and 118). In connection with the dental study, questions were asked also by the interviewers about the use of dummies or infant feeders and about the children's bedtime.

3.3.2 The dental examinations of children between the ages of 18 months and $4\frac{1}{2}$ years were carried out by local authority dental officers by arrangement with the Medical Officers of Health and Chief Dental Officers concerned. The condition of the teeth was charted and the numbers of incisor or other teeth which were either decayed, extracted or filled (def) were recorded.

3.3.3 In and around London it was possible to arrange for a medical examination to be made at the same clinic appointment by a Medical Officer of the Ministry of Health. All the examinations were made by the same doctor in order to avoid inter-observer error. Thus for practical reasons (chiefly availability of time) a smaller proportion of children was medically examined than in the pilot study. The results of these medical examinations were not included in the computer analysis, but they have been considered in the detailed study of individuals and selected groups of children.

3.4 Analysis of records

3.4.1 The fieldwork records and the results of the dental examinations were edited and coded, and the coded results recorded on punched cards for processing by computer. In the analysis of results, although the sample was not stratified by age, subjects were grouped into four age groups:

group 1: 6 months and under $1\frac{1}{2}$ years
group 2: $1\frac{1}{2}$ and under $2\frac{1}{2}$ years
group 3: $2\frac{1}{2}$ and under $3\frac{1}{2}$ years
group 4: $3\frac{1}{2}$ and under $4\frac{1}{2}$ years.

In the interpretation of results it should be borne in mind that although the youngest group spanned 6 to 18 months, two-thirds of the children in the group were over 12 months of age (para 4.7).

4. Sample response

4.1 Of the 2 321 children selected for the sample, 236 were found to be outside the scope of the survey for the following reasons:

Died	2
Moved away	142
Temporarily away	9
Not known at address	24
Still breast fed	2
At school	50
Other reasons	7

4.2 The effective sample was, therefore, 2 085 and an interview was obtained in 1 938 households. In the other 147 households either it was found impossible to make contact with the family or there were reasons for not interviewing, such as the child or parent being too ill or in hospital. Thirty-four of the mothers interviewed refused to give any information and a further 23 spoke too little English.

4.3 Complete and usable diet records were produced by 1 321 mothers or guardians in respect of 673 boys and 648 girls. The information available on the other 560 who were interviewed but did not produce a diet record has been analysed by age group, family size, social class, father's income level and other relevant socio-economic characteristics, and figures are given later in this report (Tables A4 and 5 (pp 39 and 40) and paras 5.1 to 5.4). Such differences as emerged in these respects between participants who produced and those who did not produce diet records were useful guides to ways in which the diet survey population may have been deficient or unrepresentative.

4.4 Of the 1 881 participants, 1 688 children were weighed and height was measured in 1 627 cases. These numbers include 382 and 373 respectively for whom diet records were not obtained.

4.5 The numbers of children about whom the various categories of information were obtained are set out fully in Table 4.1 together with the response rate for each category:

Table 4.1 : *Analysis of the response rate and information obtained in the survey*

No. of children	Information obtained				No information obtained		
	Socio-economic	Usable diet records	Height	Weight	Interviewed: refused to participate	Interviewed: language difficulties	Not inter-viewed
1254	✓	✓	✓	✓			
52	✓	✓		✓			
15	✓	✓					
373	✓		✓	✓			
9	✓			✓			
178	✓						
34					✓		
23						✓	
147							✓
Totals: 2085	1881	1321	1627	1688	34	23	147
Percentage of sample total	90.2	63.4	78.0	81.0	1.6	1.1	7.1

Number interviewed = 1938 (brace spanning rows 1254 to 147)

This shows that, although a dietary record was obtained for only about two-thirds of the sample (an experience not unusual in this kind of survey), useful social and background information was obtained from over 90%, and heights and weights recorded for about 80%.

4.6   Table A1 (p 38) shows the distribution by age and family size of children for whom usable dietary records were obtained and compares it with the numbers interviewed. In all, 68.2% of those interviewed produced dietary records, but the response was lower in the larger families, falling to 59.4% in families with four or more children under 15 years of age.

4.7   The age distribution was not even throughout the range of four years covered by the survey, due partly to loss of the older children who attended nursery schools, and partly to the defects of the sampling procedures which selected fewer of the very young children in the later months of the field work. (Response may also have varied between age groups, but this cannot be confirmed, as the precise ages of the sample children were not recorded.)

4.8   Table A2 (p 38) shows the age and family size distributions of the 738 children over the age of 18 months who were dentally examined and the 89 who were medically examined. A few children under that age who were examined are not included. These numbers represented 66% and 8% respectively of the children over 18 months of age from whom diet records were obtained.

4.9   The numbers of children surveyed in each quarter of the year October 1967 to September 1968 are set out by age and family size in Table A3 (p 39). Whilst the numbers dealt with in each quarter were fairly consistent, the age make-up of the sample varied between quarters, mainly because of the reduced representation of younger children in the last two quarters.

5. Social and Economic Characteristics of Participants in the Survey

5.1 Social class

Table A4 (p 39) shows the distribution of the families in the survey into four groups according to the Registrar-General's Social Classification based on the occupation of the husband—RG Classes I and II, III Non-Manual, III Manual, IV and V. Of those from whom diet records were obtained 27% were in social classes I, II and III Non-Manual. The proportion of other respondents in those social classes was significantly lower (18%) and there was, therefore, a bias in recording the diet in favour of the higher social classes. The family size and social class relationships are interesting. Approximately half the families of each size in the dietary survey were in class III Manual, but a greater proportion of the larger families were in classes IV and V (28% of those with 4 or more children against 18% of those with 1 or 2 children). Conversely, a greater proportion of the smaller families were in classes I, II and III Non-Manual (31% against 22%). The pattern was similar among those from whom social information only was obtained—32% of the larger families and 26% of the smaller families were in classes IV and V; 26% of the smaller families and 13% of the larger families were in classes I, II and III Non-Manual.

5.2 Employment of the mother

Altogether 166 (12.6%) of the mothers were in paid employment, the proportion rising, as might be expected, with the age of the child. In families with 1 or 2 children under 15 years of age, the number of working mothers rose to 17.2%. This is not necessarily a true index of the proportion of mothers of young children going out to work, since working may well have been a reason for non-response or failure by the interviewer to make contact. As might be expected, a larger proportion (20.5%) of the mothers who gave social information but not diet records were employed.

5.3 Income

5.3.1 Respondents were asked to state the usual gross weekly income of the child's father or, if there was no father, of the mother. As in the National Food Survey of the Ministry of Agriculture, Fisheries and Food, if this gross weekly income was less than £11 and another member of the household had a larger income, the latter was substituted. The distribution of incomes in family size groups is shown in Table A5 (p 40), and comparable figures from the National Food Survey, 1967 and 1968 (Ministry of Agriculture, Fisheries and

Food, 1969, 1970) are given in Table A6 (p 40). The latter includes households with members of all ages and those without children or with children outside the age range of the nutrition survey. Nevertheless, the distributions of incomes in the two surveys are not very dissimilar.

5.3.2   Of those who produced diet records, 41% earned less than £19 per week, including 2% who earned less than £11. For those who gave socio-economic information only, the corresponding figures were 53% and 4%. This indicates that the low earners were significantly under-represented among those who produced usable diet records.

5.3.3   Ninety-nine (7.5%) households where a diet record was obtained had 2 earning members, either whole or part-time, and 44 (3.3%) had 3 or more earners. The proportions were larger—12% and 4.5% respectively—in the other households about which socio-economic but not dietary information was obtained, no doubt a consequence of their including more of the larger families and working mothers.

5.3.4   It is difficult to judge whether the diet survey sample was representative from the economic point of view. The income distribution was not greatly out of line with that of respondents in the National Food Survey, but a comparison between respondents producing diet records and those who did not indicatet that children with lower-earning fathers were under-represented in the dies survey.

5.4   School leaving age of the mother

The majority of mothers finished their full-time education at or before the age of 15. Only 321 mothers (24.3%) continued their schooling after that age—27.5% of those with 1 or 2 children, 23.7% of those with 3 children and 20.4% of those with 4 or more children. The proportion was lower still (17.7%) among the mothers who did not furnish diet records, possibly because there were some whose educational standard was so poor that they were unable to understand what was required and could not compile a record.

5.5   One-parent families

The survey was not designed to make a specific study of children with only one parent in the household. In fact, in only 26 cases was the mother the only adult in the family. There were a further 18 cases where no father was reported but a grandparent or another relative of the child was living in the household as well as the mother. Together, these constituted 3.3% of the children surveyed.

5.6 Immigrant families

These, too, were not numerous enough to provide material for a separate study of intakes; 108 mothers were born in countries other than England, Scotland and Wales, but of these 92 had been resident in Great Britain for 5 years or more, 55 of them for over 10 years. Their distribution by country of origin was:

Africa	6
European countries (excluding Ireland and the UK)	11
India or Pakistan	7
Ireland (Eire and NI)	54
West Indies	24
Other countries	6

6. Food and Nutrient Intakes

6.1 Food intakes

6.1.1 *Energy*

Diagrams A1–12 (pp 68–79) show the percentages of energy and individual nutrients provided by groups of foods. Food sources of energy were very similar within age groups (para 3.4.1), showing a consistent dietary pattern. In age groups 1 and 2 the principal source of energy was milk. In the youngest age group manufactured baby foods provided 11% of the total energy and slightly more than 11% came from the group of foods including biscuits, cakes etc. The older children (age groups 3 and 4) derived 18% of total energy from biscuits, cakes etc., and about 15% from milk. The two groups of foods containing preserves and confectionery between them contributed about 13% of energy in all age groups. On the whole, the higher average energy intakes of children in larger families were associated with greater consumption of bread and flour-based foods.

6.1.2 *Protein*

Milk provided more protein than any other single food. This was true for all age groups and all family sizes, but in the two older age groups meat and meat dishes provided almost as much of the total protein as did milk.

6.1.3 *Animal protein*

In all age and family size groups the chief sources of animal protein were milk, which provided 35–50%, meat 15–30%, and eggs 10% of the total. Children in age group 4 derived 6–7% of total animal protein from fish but very little was eaten in the younger age groups and cheese consumption in all age groups was negligible. The proportion of total milk coming from dried milk (infant formula) was higher for children in small families than for those in large families. This is discussed later in relation to vitamin D intakes (para 6.1.14).

6.1.4 *Fat*

In all age groups, milk was the chief source of fat in the diet. The youngest children obtained 40% of their fat from milk (including 7% from dried milk) and the oldest 20%. As would be expected, the older children obtained more of their dietary fat from flour confectionery (cakes, biscuits, etc.), other dairy products (but not cheese to any great extent) and meat dishes.

6.1.5 *Carbohydrate*[1]

Carbohydrate provided about 50% of the total energy for children of all age groups and from all family sizes. In the youngest age group manufactured baby foods, biscuits and cakes, milk, preserves and bread were the main sources of carbohydrate. In all except the youngest age group, the pattern of food sources of carbohydrate consumption in the form of flour confectionery, bread, preserves and cereals was the same as that known from previous surveys to be characteristic of adults (Department of Health and Social Security, 1971 (unpublished); 1972).

6.1.6 *"Added sugars"*

"Added sugars" (para 3.2.3) provided on average about one-fifth of the total energy of the diet, and the food sources of these added sugars were therefore of interest. In all age groups and among children from different family sizes, the group of foods including jam, honey and other preserves was the main contributor and provided 35–48% of the total added sugars. In all age groups total consumption of added sugars was slightly higher among children in large families, and on the whole this seemed to be due to a greater intake of preserves and confectionery (sweets). Even in the youngest age group sweets provided 9% of total added sugars, but in all groups of children over $1\frac{1}{2}$ years of age more sweets were eaten and 22% of added sugars was derived from them.

6.1.7 *Calcium*

Calcium was obtained very largely from milk (including dried milk), which provided 56–67% of the total intake. In the youngest age group manufactured baby foods contributed 9% of the total intake, and in all age groups milk, bread and other foods made with flour between them provided about 78% of the total calcium intake.

6.1.8 *Iron*

The main sources of iron in the youngest age group were manufactured baby foods and cereals. Between them, these two food groups provided 50% of the total iron intake. Only 9% of the total consumption in this age group was from meat. Older children obtained 19–23% of their total iron from meat and meat dishes, 7–9% from egg and egg dishes and appreciable amounts of iron were also derived from cereals and flour-based foods.

6.1.9 *Thiamin*

Food sources of thiamin were many. As would be expected breakfast cereals, milk and flour products headed the list. The youngest children obtained 10% of total thiamin from manufactured baby foods but in the older age groups this source of thiamin was replaced by potatoes.

---

[1]Throughout the report "carbohydrate" refers to total carbohydrates and includes "added sugars".

13

6.1.10 *Riboflavin*

In all age groups the outstanding source of riboflavin (41–50%) was milk. Breakfast cereals and flour products provided another 17–20%. If milk consumption were halved, the mean intake in every age group would still satisfy the recommended daily intake (Department of Health and Social Security, 1969) even without an increase in other foods.

6.1.11 *Nicotinic acid*

The two principal sources of nicotinic acid were breakfast cereals and meat and meat dishes; these foods contributed about 40–45% of total intake in all but the youngest age group, where the contribution was between 30 and 40%. Manufactured baby foods were an important source of the vitamin in the youngest age group.

6.1.12 *Vitamin A*

Major food sources of vitamin A in all age groups were milk and liver. Fats and oils also provided appreciable amounts of this vitamin for all groups of children over $1\frac{1}{2}$ years of age and vitamin supplements were good sources below the age of $2\frac{1}{2}$ years. It is worth noting that even without the vitamin A contribution from supplements, the diet of the younger children would contain more than the recommended daily intake of vitamin A.

6.1.13 *Vitamin C*

The percentage of the total vitamin C intake which derived from fortified manufactured baby foods and vitamin supplements varied from 18% (children over $3\frac{1}{2}$ years in families of 4 or more) to 64% (children under $1\frac{1}{2}$ years in families of less than 3). It is apparent that without these fortified foods and supplements average intakes would, in many cases, be below recommended levels. Most of the children received proprietary brands of vitamin supplements; the uptake of welfare supplements was very small. The contribution of potatoes to the vitamin C intake varied from 30% (children over $3\frac{1}{2}$ years in families of 4 or more) to 8% (children under $1\frac{1}{2}$ years in families of 3 or less). Similarly a larger contribution from raw and citrus fruits was found in the older than in the younger children. In all age groups potatoes were a larger source of vitamin C in the diet than fresh fruit.

6.1.14 *Vitamin D*

In no group of children did the vitamin D intake reach recommended levels. Highest average intakes were found for children in small families in the youngest age group. These children obtained about 75% of their total intake from fortified milks, manufactured baby foods and vitamin supplements. As consumption of these foods and vitamin supplements declined so did total intake, dropping from a maximum of 261 iu (6.5 µg) for children under $1\frac{1}{2}$ years in

14

families of less than 3, to a minimum of 66 iu (1.7 µg) for children over $3\frac{1}{2}$ years in families of 3. The older children did not fully make up for this loss by eating enough of the limited number of foods naturally containing this vitamin.

6.1.15 *Principal animal protein contributing foods*

An analysis of the intake of certain important *foods* (milk, meat, egg, fish, cheese) by individuals showed the total amount of each food consumed per day, whether the food was eaten as such or as part of a composite item, for example, meat in a meat pie or milk in a milk pudding. Diagrams A13 and 14 (pp 80 and 81) give the range of intakes of milk and meat respectively for the different age groups. The intakes of egg, fish and cheese were consistently small —the ranges of the daily intakes of these foods through the four age groups were 0.8–0.9 oz egg, 0.1–0.3 oz fish and 0.0–0.1 oz cheese per child.

6.2 Seasonal variation of intakes

6.2.1 The histograms in Diagram A15 (p 82) show the mean energy intakes of the four age groups of survey children for the four separate three-month periods of the year. The intakes in the coldest quarter as shown by recorded air temperature (January–March) gave a slightly higher average than those in the warmest quarter (July–September). The mean intakes of protein, carbohydrate and fat followed this pattern but the differences were small and not significant. Seasonal variations of vitamin C were not assessed as it was impossible to get the accurate information about place of origin, length of storage etc., which would be needed for accurate coding. Consequently, a weighted average figure for vitamin C content was used in the food composition table for those fruits and vegetables which are known to have significant seasonal variations.

6.3 Nutrient intakes

6.3.1 The mean daily intake of nutrients and of the percentage of energy derived from protein, fat and "added sugars" (para 3.2.3) are given for the separate age groups and family sizes in Tables A7–10 (pp 41–44) inclusive, and the frequency distributions of mean daily intakes during the week of study for energy and some nutrients are shown in Diagrams A16–23 (pp 83–90) inclusive. As in the pilot study, there was a wide range in mean intakes of each individual nutrient.

6.3.2 In all groups the mean daily intakes of energy, total protein, fat, carbohydrate and "added sugars" rose with age. Calcium intake on the other hand fell with age, as did the average intake of milk. Iron intake dropped considerably after the age of $1\frac{1}{2}$ years, but rose again after $3\frac{1}{2}$ years of age. The intakes of vitamins A, D and C were also highest in the youngest age groups among whom vitamin supplements would most likely be included in the diet. The percentage of energy derived from protein was also highest in the youngest age group and fell with age.

6.3.3 Table A11 (p 45) shows the recommended daily intakes of energy and nutrients for children of different age groups (Department of Health and Social Security, 1969). When comparing the mean daily intakes of groups of children in the survey with these recommended intakes, allowance has to be made for the fact that the age spans of the groups of children in this survey are not identical with those in the report of the pilot study (Ministry of Health, 1968). In addition there were relatively few children under 12 months of age (para 4.7).

6.3.4 The energy intake of each individual child was compared with the intake recommended for the particular age of that child and 850 of the 1 321 children studied (64%) had energy intakes below the recommended level for their age. These included 391 (58%) boys (Diagram A.24(a), p 91) and 462 (71%) girls (Diagram A24(b), p 91). This was an interesting result both from a statistical and from a nutritional point of view, and is discussed later (para 10.3.1).

6.3.5 The figures given in Tables A7–10 (pp 41–44) indicate that the mean intakes of protein and the percentages of energy obtained from protein in all age and family size groups were above the appropriate recommended levels. Mean intakes of calcium, vitamins A and C, riboflavin and thiamin were all well above those recommended. The mean intake of iron barely reached the recommended level and that of vitamin D fell considerably short of it. However a dietary intake of vitamin D takes no account of the synthesis of this vitamin by the action of ultraviolet light on the skin, and the amount synthesized cannot easily be quantified. The recommended intake for nicotinic acid is expressed as nicotinic acid equivalents, i.e. allowing for the conversion of tryptophan to nicotinic acid in the body. The food tables used in this survey however do not provide for nicotinic acid to be expressed as "equivalents" since the tryptophan content of many foods has not yet been estimated. Thus nicotinic acid is calculated from the food tables as mg of the vitamin. In the 1968 National Food Survey the tryptophan content of the diet was assumed to be approximately 1.4% of the animal protein consumed (Paul, 1969) and it is unlikely to be less in the protein of the pre-school child's diet. Using this approximation to calculate the nicotinic acid equivalents of the diet, the mean intake for all the age/family size groups was well above the recommended intake.

6.3.6 In comparing the mean daily intake of nutrients in the children from families of different size, it can be seen that the intakes of energy, fat, carbohydrate and "added sugars" were significantly greater in subjects where there were 4 or more children in the family and, as indicated in para 6.1.1, this was eaten in the form of bread and other flour-based foods. In the two youngest age groups protein intakes were unrelated to size of family, but in the two oldest groups children in the larger families consumed more protein than children in small families, the difference being in protein of non-animal origin. In the youngest age group children in small families did better for iron than those in large families, but in the two oldest age groups the situation was reversed. No relationship was found between calcium intakes and family size. In all age groups the intake of vitamin C fell as the size of the family grew, and in the youngest age groups the intake of vitamin D was less in the larger families.

6.3.7   Children from families in social classes IV and V had mean daily intakes of energy, total protein, fat, carbohydrate, calcium and iron higher than those of children from social classes I and II (Table A12, p 46). The percentage of energy from protein and fat were lower in social classes IV and V. The intakes of vitamins A, C and D were however smaller in the children from social classes IV and V. The only nutrient for which there was a pronounced social class gradient was vitamin C, and the intakes of this vitamin were considerably smaller in social classes IV and V in all family size groups (Table A13, p 47).

6.3.8   Table A14 (p 48) shows mean daily nutrient intakes of children according to the income of the "father" as defined in para 5.3.1. Except for energy and carbohydrate, the children whose fathers earned less than £19 per week had lower intakes than those whose fathers earned more, and this was markedly so for vitamins A, C and D and for iron. In the 31 cases where the income was less than £11 (23 of them fatherless children) protein, fat, calcium, riboflavin and nicotinic acid intakes were also lower. These children will be considered later (para 9.4). An interesting finding was that children whose fathers had the biggest incomes (£32 or more per week) had smaller intakes of energy, and ate less of "added sugars", but they obtained a slightly higher percentage of energy from protein. They also had substantially higher intakes of vitamins A, C and D.

6.3.9   The mean daily intakes of energy, carbohydrate and "added sugars" were lower (the two last to a statistically significant extent), and those of all other nutrients higher, in children whose mothers stayed at school after the age of 15 (Table A15, p 49). Differences in intake where the mother was in paid employment were not so marked. The differences in energy intake were statistically significant—the children of working mothers averaging some 70 kcal (0.29 MJ) more than the children of non-working mothers. They also had slightly higher intakes of protein, fat and "added sugars", but less of vitamins A, C and D (Table A15, p 49).

6.4   Comparison with the Bransby and Fothergill survey of 1951 and with the pilot survey of 1963

6.4.1   A comparison of the mean nutrient intakes in this survey with those in the 1963 pilot survey (Ministry of Health, 1968), and with the survey of Bransby and Fothergill (1954) is shown in Table A16 (p 50). Although the pilot survey involved a smaller sample of children from fewer areas in only one season of the year, the most interesting feature of the comparison is the compatibility of the 1963 and 1967–68 results. There are differences, notably that the "added sugars" and total carbohydrate mean intakes were higher in 1967–68 for all age groups, as were also the intakes of nicotinic acid and vitamin C, and that in all except the youngest group the intake of vitamin D was lower.

The mean daily intake of iron in all but the oldest group was lower in the 1967–68 survey than in the 1963 pilot survey, and failed to reach the recommended levels in all but the youngest group. However, intakes of meat from all sources per 1 000 kcal were slightly higher in the later survey; intakes of other iron-containing foods, for example bread, were the same, and of eggs and egg dishes only slightly lower. A higher proportion of children in large families was intentionally included in the 1967–68 survey. Because of this and the different age ranges in the two surveys, comparison of intakes cannot be exact (para 6.3.3).

6.4.2 The Bransby and Fothergill survey involved 461 children in 10 areas in April 1951, and in these respects resembled the pilot survey more closely; but the methodology and food composition tables were different and food rationing was still in force. The results of the 1951 survey on the whole are out of line with those of the more recent surveys and usually show higher intakes.

6.5 Summary of results

6.5.1 Broadly speaking these results show that the mean nutrient intakes of the groups of children in this survey, whether classified by age, number of children in the family, social class or income of the head of the household, compare favourably with the recommended daily intakes of the Department of Health and Social Security (1969).

6.5.2 Children in small families and those in social classes I and II and in groups where the mother's education was continued after 15 years of age in general had a diet in which the mean daily intakes of fat and "added sugars" were less, but of vitamin C and sometimes of other vitamins greater, than children in larger families, in social classes IV and V, and whose mothers left school at 15 years of age or before.

7. Heights and weights

7.1 Measurements

7.1.1 The height of the child at the time of the survey was recorded in 1 627 cases, and the weight in 1 688 cases (para 4.4). Heights of all children were measured in the supine position (Appendix C). A comparison was made between children with and without diet records in respect of weight and height distributions. There was no significant or consistent difference between them in any age group.

7.1.2 Height was not measured in 13.5% of the children. Measurement was found to be easiest in the youngest children and most difficult in those aged $1\frac{1}{2}$ and under $2\frac{1}{2}$ years. Weights were obtained in a slightly higher proportion of children; only 10.3% were not weighed, the figure increasing with the age of the child. Response for the girls was about 3% better than for the boys for both measurements (Table 7.1.).

Table 7.1: *Percentage of children in the different age groups who were not measured or weighed*

	All children	Age group (years)			
		$\frac{1}{2}$ and under $1\frac{1}{2}$	$1\frac{1}{2}$ and under $2\frac{1}{2}$	$2\frac{1}{2}$ and under $3\frac{1}{2}$	$3\frac{1}{2}$ and under $4\frac{1}{2}$
Height	13.5	10.6	15.0	13.7	13.2
Weight	10.3	8.1	9.4	11.0	11.7

7.1.3 The response was better among the children for whom diet records were produced. Only 5.1% failed to have their heights measured and 1.1% failed to be weighed.

7.2 Parents' heights

The fathers' and mothers' heights were also obtained in 1 210 cases. A regression analysis between the children's and the individual parents' heights revealed significant relationships with the mother's height in 7 of the 8 age/sex groups and with the father's height in 3 of the 8 groups. As the age of the child increased there was no evidence of any decrease in the importance of the height of either parent as a factor in determining the height of the child. There was no conclusive evidence of a child's height being more dependent on the height of the parent of the same sex than on the height of the parent of the opposite sex.

7.3 Adjustment of heights and weights for age

In relating stature to energy and nutrient intakes and to socio-economic factors it was necessary to eliminate age variations within the range of 12 months in each age group. For each child for whom there was a diet record an adjusted height and weight were calculated. This was standardized to the midpoint of the age range by reference to normal rates of growth (Tanner, Whitehouse and Takaishi, 1966). The means and standard deviations of the adjusted heights of boys and girls in each age group are shown in Table 7.2, and the frequency distributions of the adjusted heights and weights are given in Diagrams A25(a)–(d) (p 92) and A26(a)–(d) (p 93) respectively. Most of these distributions were approximately normal (i.e. symmetrical and Gaussian) and were not, therefore significantly skewed, but in age group 3 the heights of boys and girls were a little more widely distributed below the median than they were above it.

Table 7.2: *Mean heights and weights (adjusted for age) of pre-school children in the different age/sex groups*

Age group (years)	Height			Weight		
	Number of children	Mean cm	S.D.[1]	Number of children	Mean kg	S.D.[1]
BOYS						
$\frac{1}{2}$ and under $1\frac{1}{2}$	103	75.7	4.58	104	10.9	1.4
$1\frac{1}{2}$ and under $2\frac{1}{2}$	186	85.9	4.08	200	12.9	1.5
$2\frac{1}{2}$ and under $3\frac{1}{2}$	188	94.3	5.35	195	14.7	1.8
$3\frac{1}{2}$ and under $4\frac{1}{2}$	164	101.7	5.04	167	16.5	2.0
GIRLS						
$\frac{1}{2}$ and under $1\frac{1}{2}$	96	73.5	3.68	99	9.9	1.4
$1\frac{1}{2}$ and under $2\frac{1}{2}$	181	84.9	3.83	194	12.2	1.5
$2\frac{1}{2}$ and under $3\frac{1}{2}$	194	92.8	4.89	200	13.9	1.8
$3\frac{1}{2}$ and under $4\frac{1}{2}$	142	100.4	4.72	147	16.0	1.9

[1] S.D. = Standard deviation.

7.4 Socio-economic factors affecting height

7.4.1 Tables A17–24 (pp 51–54) show the percentage distribution of boys and girls according to their heights (adjusted for age), by the number of children under 15 years of age in the household, social class, the income of the head of the household and by the age at which the mother left school. In this survey height tended to fall with increasing size of family, but significant relationships (P=0.05) were found only in the girls (except those in the youngest age group); they were not found in boys of any age. In the oldest age group of girls, height was significantly related to social class (P=0.02), classes I, II and III Non-Manual being taller than the other classes. In the boys and other age groups of girls there was no relationship between height and social class. In two groups only—age group 1 boys and age group 3 girls—height and income of father were related (P=0.05), the children of fathers earning £19 per week or more being significantly taller than the children of those earning less than that sum. A positive relationship between height and the age at which the mother left school

20

was found in only one group—age group 4 boys— and then only to a marginally significant degree (P=0.10).

7.4.2   The mean Quetelet's index[1] for boys and girls in the different age groups was calculated using heights and weights adjusted for age, and was found to fall with increasing age in both sexes, and to be smaller for girls in the three younger age groups (Table 7.3.).

Table 7.3: *Mean Quetelet's index in children of different ages*

Sex	Age group (years)			
	$\frac{1}{2}$ and under 1$\frac{1}{2}$	1$\frac{1}{2}$ and under 2$\frac{1}{2}$	2$\frac{1}{2}$ and under 3$\frac{1}{2}$	3$\frac{1}{2}$ and under 4$\frac{1}{2}$
Boys	1.9	1.8	1.7	1.6
Girls	1.8	1.7	1.6	1.6

7.5   Nutrient intakes and anthropometry

7.5.1   Although the number of children who refused measurements of height and weight was small, a comparison of the percentage of their energy intake from protein was made for the two groups. Only 15 children refused to be weighed and their mean percentage of energy from protein was the same (11.9%) as that of the 1 306 children who were weighed. The 67 children whose heights were not measured obtained 11.6% of their energy from protein compared with 11.9% for the 1 254 children who were measured. This difference is not significant.

7.5.2   Tables A25 and 26 (pp 55 and 56) set out the mean energy and protein intakes for children of different heights and weights in each age group. Regression analysis produced no clear evidence that differences in intake of protein were associated with variations in height or weight. There was however evidence of a direct relationship of energy intake with height and weight: a difference of 100 kcal (0.418 MJ) was associated in the boys aged 6 months and under 1$\frac{1}{2}$ years with 0.89 cm difference in height, and in the girls aged 3$\frac{1}{2}$ and under 4$\frac{1}{2}$ years with 0.65 kg difference in weight; there were lesser differences in the other age/sex groups. Except for the youngest age group of boys, Quetelet's index increased fairly consistently with intakes of both energy and protein but not with protein per 1 000 kcal (Table A27, p 57). There was no relationship between Quetelet's index and the intakes of either carbohydrate or "added sugars".

7.5.3   A further analysis was made within social class and family size groups relating weight to mean intakes of energy, total protein, fat, carbohydrate and "added sugars". Intakes of these nutrients were found to be higher in large families and in those from social classes IV and V (paras 6.3.6 and 6.3.7), but the analysis did not reveal any consistent weight pattern.

[1]Quetelet's index is defined as $\frac{\text{weight (kg)}}{\text{height (cm)}^2} \times 1000$ (Kemsley, Billewicz and Thomson, 1962).

8. Heights and weights in relation to milk consumption

8.1 All children were entitled under the Welfare Foods scheme at the time of the survey to one pint of cheap liquid milk daily or the equivalent 20 oz dried milk powder per week. The "take-up" of welfare milk tokens among the 1 321 families participating was almost 100%, but the mean daily intake of milk drunk by the survey children during the week of the dietary record varied widely in all age groups, and there was a very high percentage of children taking less than their full pint of liquid milk per day, the percentage increasing with age. It can only be concluded that much of this "Welfare" milk was consumed by other members of the family.

Table 8.1: *Percentage of children with milk intake of less than 20 oz per day*

Age group	Percentage
6 mth and under $1\frac{1}{2}$ yr	76
$1\frac{1}{2}$ yr and under $2\frac{1}{2}$ yr	89
$2\frac{1}{2}$ yr and under $3\frac{1}{2}$ yr	93
$3\frac{1}{2}$ yr and under $4\frac{1}{2}$ yr	95

8.2 An analysis of the average daily intake of milk from all sources by different socio-economic factors showed that there was no evidence of milk consumption being affected by family size, social class or the age at which the mother left school. For each of these factors there was no consistent difference and not even any difference in the same direction. An association was found between milk intake and very low income (the under £11 group averaging 2.5 oz less than the others) but the relationship did not persist above that level.

8.3 Milk is an important food for younger children since 1 pint of it supplies 380 kcal (1.58 MJ) energy, 18 g protein, 680 mg calcium and 0.76 mg riboflavin. Table A28 (p 58) shows the contribution made by milk to the intakes of these nutrients. Within the different age groups the mean daily intakes of energy and the three nutrients were compared for the children below the 25th percentile for total milk intake with the intakes for those above the 75th percentile (Tables A29–32, pp 58–60). The range of milk intake was wide, the average amount of milk drunk by children in the upper quartile being 2½ to 3 times that drunk by children in the lowest quartile. Comparison with the recommended daily intakes shown in Table A11 (p 45) indicates that, in all age and family size groups, the intake of riboflavin was adequate even for the group which drank least milk, but that that of calcium was not. The shortfall was small but apparently the children who drank little milk did not replace the milk by other sources of calcium in sufficient quantity to reach the level of the recommended intake. The protein intakes of these children were just below those recommended only in the older groups aged $2\frac{1}{2}$ and under $3\frac{1}{2}$ years, and $3\frac{1}{2}$ and under $4\frac{1}{2}$ years. Only in the youngest group of those who drank least milk was the recommended energy intake reached; in this survey 64% of the children had energy intakes below those recommended (paras 6.3.4 and 10.3.1).

8.4 In the report of the pilot survey of pre-school children (Ministry of Health, 1968) p 72 carries the statement: "The heights and weights of all children who were weighed and measured have been averaged for those falling in each quarter in respect of milk consumption. Though the numbers involved are far too small to be convincing, there appears to be a relationship at least between height and milk consumption. Whether this relationship, if real, is causal is another matter". Accordingly an analysis of the results of the 1967–68 survey was made to find out if they too showed a relationship between height and/or weight and milk intake.

8.5 Individual milk intakes were plotted against the age of the child in days. The scatter indicated that there was no relationship between the two in this study, and hence actual milk intakes were used in the analysis. Tables A33 and 34 (pp 60 and 61) show the heights and weights of boys and girls separately according to the different quartiles of total milk intake. All heights were adjusted to the mid-point of the age group (para 7.3). Although in most groups there was a tendency for height to increase with milk intake, the tendency was only slight and not consistent. Even in the lowest age group, in which for many children milk was the predominant item of diet, the differences were very small and, in the case of the girls, in the reverse direction. The differences in weights, although not entirely consistent, were rather more marked, particularly in the boys.

8.6 A simple regression analysis revealed a significant relationship (P=0.05) between height and milk intake only for boys aged $1\frac{1}{2}$ and under $2\frac{1}{2}$ years. In spite of the much larger sample of children surveyed compared with the pilot survey, the analysis under discussion still involved relatively small numbers in the individual groups. In addition, growth is not solely dependent on nutrition, but may be affected by other environmental factors, and any relationship between height and milk intake may therefore have been coincidental.

9. Special groups of children

9.1 Children with low intakes of milk

9.1.1 Twenty children (5 in each age group—8 boys and 12 girls) with the lowest milk intake were found to have intakes varying from 0.55 to 4.98 oz per day compared with means ranging, for the youngest to the oldest age groups, from 16.2 to 12.0 oz per day. The children were from families of all sizes and social classes and were found to have intakes, not only of the three main nutrients in milk but also of total energy, which were low in relation to age group means. They also obtained a smaller proportion of energy from protein (Table 9.1).

Table 9.1: *Mean intakes of some nutrients of 20 children (5 in each age group) who drank the least amount of milk, compared with average nutrient intakes of all the children*

Age group (years)	Children	Energy kcal/MJ	Total protein g	Energy from protein %	Calcium mg	Riboflavin mg
½ and under 1½	All	1050/4.4	33.9	13.0	771	1.25
	Low milk	961/4.0	25.7	11.0	419	0.80
1½ and under 2½	All	1262/5.3	38.0	12.1	691	1.07
	Low milk	890/3.7	21.7	9.7	286	0.49
2½ and under 3½	All	1401/5.9	40.7	11.7	658	1.07
	Low milk	1202/5.0	28.6	9.7	291	0.52
3½ and under 4½	All	1468/6.1	41.6	11.4	661	1.08
	Low milk	1306/5.5	33.9	10.5	315	0.70

9.1.2 The five youngest children were all shorter and lighter in weight than average; the five oldest children were all taller than average, four being heavier and one lighter in weight than average.

9.2 Children with high intakes of "added sugars"

9.2.1 The five children in each age group with the highest daily intake of "added sugars" were found to be 13 boys and 7 girls, predominantly from large families of social classes III Manual, IV and V.

9.2.2 These children ate daily an amount of "added sugars" which was more than twice the mean intake for their age group. Sweets, biscuits, cakes and jam figured prominently in their diet, but sweetened drinks (tea, coffee, milk and squashes) made a large contribution.

9.2.3 Their intakes of carbohydrate, energy and protein were higher, and the percentage of energy derived from protein was less than the age group mean.

9.2.4 The majority of the children (12) were below or the same as the mean weight for their age/sex group, and 6 of the 8 who were heavier than average were also taller. There was thus little evidence from this small group of children that a high consumption of "added sugars" was associated with overweight.

9.2.5 Dental evidence of any relationship between a high intake of "added sugars" and the number of teeth which are decayed, extracted or filled (def) was incomplete. Of the 20 children under consideration, 14 were not dentally examined, 3 had teeth in good condition, 2 (age group 4) had 6 and 8 "def" teeth respectively, and one (age group 2) had one "def" tooth (Appendix E).

9.3 Children with low energy intakes

9.3.1 The 10% of children with the lowest energy intake for each age group were considered individually. There were 58 boys and 75 girls. All family sizes, social classes and income groups were represented among the families of these children.

9.3.2 Table A35 (p 62) compares the mean daily intakes of energy and some nutrients of these children with the intakes for the whole group under study. Although the intakes of energy, protein, carbohydrate and "added sugars" were lower, the percentage of energy derived from these nutrients was not significantly different in these children when compared with all the survey children.

Table 9.2: *The mean heights and weights of the 10% of children[1] with the lowest energy intakes compared with those of the other 90% in the different age/sex groups (numbers in parentheses)*

Age group (years)	Height in cm		Weight in kg	
	Lowest 10% energy intake	Other 90%	Lowest 10% energy intake	Other 90%
BOYS				
½ and under 1½	75.2 (12)	75.8 (91)	10.2 (12)	11.0 (92)
1½ and under 2½	86.5 (16)	85.8 (170)	12.4 (16)	12.9 (184)
2½ and under 3½	93.3 (18)	94.4 (170)	14.1 (18)	14.8 (177)
3½ and under 4½	101.2 (11)	101.7 (153)	15.7 (11)	16.6 (156)
GIRLS				
½ and under 1½	73.5 (8)	73.5 (88)	9.9 (8)	9.9 (90)
1½ and under 2½	85.2 (20)	84.9 (161)	11.9 (23)	12.2 (171)
2½ and under 3½	90.8 (20)	93.0 (174)	12.9 (20)	14.0 (180)
3½ and under 4½	100.2 (21)	100.4 (121)	15.2 (22)	16.1 (125)

[1] One boy was not weighed or measured, six girls were not measured and two girls were not weighed.

25

9.3.3 The individual case records were scrutinized in an attempt to find some explanation for the low energy intake, although the questionnaire was not designed specifically to elicit this. In all age groups over 50% of these children were said by the mother to have been unwell (teething troubles and minor illnesses) for the week of the survey, and in the youngest age group the figure reached 65%. Some case records reported food "fads", and some domestic crises of one sort or another during the week of the survey. There may have been some association between these alleged conditions and the reduced energy intake. For about 40% of children there was no recorded information which could explain it.

9.3.4 In 7 of the 8 age/sex groups, the differences between the mean height of these children and the mean height of the other 90% of survey children were 1% or less (either shorter or taller). Only the girls of age group 3 were on average $2\frac{1}{2}\%$ shorter than the rest of their age group.

9.3.5 There was a clear tendency for the low energy consumers to be lighter than the rest except for the girls in age group 1. In the other age/sex groups the mean weights of these children differed from the mean weights of the other 90% of children by amounts varying from 3 to 8% (Table 9.2).

9.4 Children from low income families

9.4.1 There were 31 children in families for whom the recorded income of the head of the household was less than £11 per week. Of these 23 are recorded as having no father in the household; 1 father had died, 4 had deserted the wife, and the parents of 7 children were separated or divorced. There was no information about 2 of the fathers, and 9 mothers were unmarried. In the 8 two-parent families, 4 fathers were in low paid employment (2 farm workers, a student and a trainee plasterer), 3 were sick and 1 was unemployed.

9.4.2 Some of these 31 children had low nutrient intakes. These intakes were compared with those of the rest of the survey children who also had low intakes. For this purpose a low level was set at an arbitrary level of about 80% of the mean intake of all children in the survey in each age group. The results, summarized in Table 9.3, show little difference between the 31 and the others for energy, total protein and iron. For vitamin C a smaller proportion of the 31 had low intakes, but for riboflavin the proportion was larger than in the rest of the children.

9.4.3 Three children had intakes which were below the arbitrary level for all the listed nutrients, and were 1–3 cm shorter than the mean heights for their age groups. They were not below average weight. None of the three was reported ill during the survey.

9.4.4 Only 28 of the 31 children were weighed and measured. Their heights and weights were not significantly different from the means for their age/sex groups. Nine boys and 7 girls were under the average height for their age and 5 boys and 7 girls were over it. The weights showed a similar pattern. Eight boys and 7 girls had a Quetelet's index lower than (or equal to) the average and 6 boys and 7 girls a higher index.

Table 9.3: *Percentage of the children from 31 low income families, and of children from other families with nutrient intakes below 80% of the mean intake for their age group*

Nutrient	Low income families %	Low income families Number	Other families %	Other families Number
Energy	23	7	22	284
Total protein	29	9	26	330
Iron	29	9	29	371
Riboflavin	48	15	38	448
Vitamin C	45	14	56	726

9.4.5 The individual case histories of those children whose intake of all except 1 or 2 nutrients was below the arbitrary level were examined, but no cause for the low intakes could be deduced.

9.5 Small children

The energy and protein intakes of the 10% of children with the smallest height, weight and Quetelet's index respectively were compared with the intakes of all children in each age and sex group (Tables A36 and A37, pp 63 and 64). The findings are not consistent throughout the groups. The shorter children had lower than average intakes of energy and protein in four groups (age groups 1, 3 and 4 boys, and age group 3 girls), but the reverse was the case in the other four groups. In respect of weight, the lighter children mostly consumed less than average, though in age group 4 (girls) intakes were substantially greater than average. As might be expected, Quetelet's index showed a more consistent relationship. The group of children with Quetelet's index below the 10th percentile had intakes of energy, protein, carbohydrate and "added sugars" about the same as or less than the average for all children (Table A38, p 65). The effect on height and weight of milk consumption was studied in some detail (Section 8).

9.6 Obese children

A study of obesity was not made in all the survey children. Only 8% were medically examined and in these no measurements were made of skinfold thickness. The intakes of energy, protein, carbohydrate and "added sugars" for the children with the highest 10% Quetelet's index were compared with the intakes of these nutrients by all the children in the different age and sex groups (Table A38, p 65). In boys aged $1\frac{1}{2}$ years and over and in girls aged 6–18 months the intakes of these nutrients were markedly greater than the means for all children. In the younger boys, and in girls of other age groups, the intakes of these nutrients were either almost the same or in some groups markedly less than for all children, e.g. carbohydrate and "added sugars" intakes in girls aged $1\frac{1}{2}$ and under $2\frac{1}{2}$ years, and $2\frac{1}{2}$ and under $3\frac{1}{2}$ years.

10. Discussion

10.1 The sample

10.1.1 This survey was probably the last occasion on which a national sample could be drawn from welfare milk registers, because the registers are now kept on a national and not on a local basis and relate only to a minority of children. The effective sample for each family size group was nationally representative of Britain and although full dietary information was obtained on only two-thirds of the sample, something is known about nearly all of the children. About 7% of the sample were not contacted for one reason or another (para 4.2); illness of a parent or of the child accounted for much of the 7% and may not have led to any serious bias in the sample, but this may not be true of other reasons for not contacting the remainder of the 7%. The overt refusal rate of about 1.6% was commendably low, as was the 1.1% in whom insuperable language barriers were encountered.

10.1.2 Of the 1 938 households interviewed, only about 12% failed to produce a usable dietary record or refused a measurement of the height or weight of the child. It is gratifying that so much was learnt about so high a proportion of the sample. The dietary intakes of those who were and were not measured were not, in any age/sex group, consistently or statistically significantly different, and neither were the heights and weights of those for whom dietary intakes were or were not recorded (para 7.1.1).

10.1.3 Nevertheless this gradual erosion of the sample which resulted in a final response rate of 63.4% for those who participated fully in the survey (para 4.5) involves the possibility of some bias in terms of the worst getting away, and the extent to which this is true is discussed fully in Section 5. The absence of demonstrable nutritional bias arising out of the comparisons cited above offers some reassurance of the general validity of the results.

10.1.4 The stratification of the sample has been described (para 2.1.2). Since height was one of the most important pieces of information obtained, it may be asked why no preliminary stratification was made by height. The answer is that the prime cause of differences in height is genetic and not environmental. One of the aims of the survey was to find out whether there was any relationship between diet and height, if possible within groups of a sort and size in which genetic influences were likely to be either non-existent or negligible.

10.2 Food and nutrient intakes

10.2.1 As would be expected, the range of individual intakes of different foods and food groups, and therefore of nutrients, was very wide, and the

28

histograms (Diagrams A1–12, pp 68–79) and scatter diagrams (Diagrams A24(a) and (b) p 91) show substantial variations both from the median and the mean, which are partly, but not wholly, due to differences in the amount of food eaten. All else being equal, the bigger the child the more food he will need and this accounts for some of the variations. Another cause of variations in the amount of food eaten, as estimated in the survey, is that for some children consumption may vary from week to week, particularly if they happen to be off colour, when they may eat less food, or if they are recovering from an indisposition, when they may well eat more. The magnitude of these (and some other) effects is indicated by the spread of values for energy intake (Diagrams A24(a) and (b), p 91).

10.2.2 But in the case of nutrients, differences in dietary pattern also had an important effect. These differences may be transient, due for example to some temporary indisposition or fad, or permanent, when they reflect social or economic status or the efficiency of the mother as a housewife. Some idea of the effect of differences in dietary pattern as opposed to the amount of food eaten may be seen by comparing the spread of values for individual intakes of nutrients with the spread of intakes of energy. The coefficients of variation of energy intake and of the intakes of certain nutrients are given in Table 10.1. Those of iron, riboflavin and vitamins C and D are substantially greater than those of protein and calcium, and reflect differences in the amount of certain rich sources of these nutrients which were fed to the children during the week of the survey.

Table 10.1 : *Co-efficients of variation of the average daily intakes of energy and some nutrients of groups of children of different ages*

Age group (years)	Energy	Protein	Calcium	Iron	Vitamin C	Vitamin D	Ribo-flavin
½ and under 1½	0.240	0.248	0.305	0.513	0.660	0.981	0.669
1½ and under 2½	0.252	0.263	0.356	0.396	0.943	1.507	0.353
2½ and under 3½	0.257	0.295	0.322	0.383	0.870	1.326	0.359
3½ and under 4½	0.257	0.303	0.332	0.305	0.859	1.326	0.346

10.2.3 The average intakes of most nutrients, but not of energy (para 10.3.1), reached or exceeded recommended levels. The exceptions (para 6.3.5.) were vitamin D and iron. In the pilot study of 1963 the large number of children with intakes of iron that were below recommended levels led to a special study by McWilliam (Ministry of Health, 1968, Appendix H) of haemoglobin levels, but the study revealed little or no anaemia and a comparable study was not repeated during the course of this survey.

10.2.4 The youngest children of all social classes and family sizes obtained most of their vitamin D, excluding that synthesized in the body as a result of

29

exposure to ultraviolet light, from fortified foods and vitamin supplements. Supplements continued to be given to the older children, chiefly in small families, in families of social classes I and II and in better off families. The older children in larger and poorer families and those from social classes IV and V mostly did not continue to receive vitamin supplements, and did not fully make up for this loss by eating more of the limited number of foods naturally containing this vitamin (paras 6.1.14 and 6.3.5).

10.2.5 There was a consistent gradient in the average intakes of vitamin C which showed a falling intake with the growing number of children per family and with a fall in income and lower social class rating; in children of all family sizes, all income groups and all social classes the mean intake was never below the recommended intake for the particular age group (para 6.3.7). In the 1963 pilot survey no relationship was found between vitamin C intake and gingivitis or any other manifestation of deficiency of this vitamin, and no indication of vitamin C deficiency was observed among the limited number of children who were medically examined in the present survey.

10.3 Energy intakes

10.3.1 The finding that 64% of the children in this survey were recorded as taking less, as opposed to more, than the recommended daily intake of energy (para 6.3.4. and Diagrams A24 (a) and (b), p 91), raises the question whether a proportion of children were undernourished and, if they were not, whether the level of the recommended daily intake of energy is set too high. Analysis showed that the average daily intake of energy is greater in children from larger families and also greater in children from social classes IV and V compared with those from social classes I and II, although they were on average no heavier (paras 6.3.6, 6.3.7 and 7.5.3; Tables A12 and 14, pp 46 and 48). Thus, low intakes of energy are inversely related to social and economic status, and the findings in this study in no way lead to the conclusion that the children with low intakes were undernourished. On the contrary, the results suggest that the level of the recommended daily intake of energy in young children may need to be re-evaluated. The requirements of an individual for energy are determined by his activity, and in health the consumption of energy is closely related to requirement. It could be that the children in large families play more together. In addition, the tendency to smaller families, and other aspects of modern life which might apply more to social classes I and II than to social classes IV and V, may be associated with a diminished physical activity of children.

10.3.2 All else being equal, the bigger the child the more energy he expends, and the relationships between energy intake and height and weight noted in para 7.5.2 are in accord with expectation. A more useful comparison is probably obtained by means of Quetelet's index (footnote, p 21), which provides a measure of weight for height which, at any age, is largely independent of the differences in height, although individuals with low and high Quetelet values may differ not only because of differences in "leanness-fatness" but also in the extent to which the body build is slender or square. The relationship between Quetelet's index and energy (and total protein) intake had to be studied with this in mind and it is pertinent that no relationship was found between Quetelet's index and the amount of protein per unit of energy; but, as expected, the energy intake increased with increasing values for Quetelet's index in all age/sex groups (Table A27, p 57).

10.4   Stature

10.4.1 Analysis of the height of the children in relation to the height of the parents showed that, as the age of the child increased, there was no evidence that the height of the parent as a factor in determining the height of the child became less important (para 7.2). No support can be adduced, from the results of this survey, for the possibility that the mother's height may influence that of her daughter more closely than that of her son, nor that the father's height may influence that of his son more closely than that of his daughter.

10.4.2 In para 7.4.1 small differences are noted between the mean stature of groups of children of different social or economic circumstances, though few of them are statistically significant. To establish any statistical significance larger numbers of children would have had to be measured in some groups. In general the findings favour a hypothesis that the better the social situation the larger the child. It is possible that the socio-economic differences which are found when children are measured at age 5 years (Scottish Home and Health Department, 1972, personal communication) or at age 7 years (Davie, Butler and Goldstein, 1972) could be shown to begin as early as the second year of life, given samples of adequate size. The differences in stature are not necessarily nutritional in origin. They could also be due to some non-nutritional factor, either genetic or environmental. It is difficult to see how this question can be resolved except by means of an investigation of a different kind from that described in this report.

10.4.3. The pilot survey in 1963 revealed a possible relationship between height and milk consumption. Because of this possibility, and because of the changes in Welfare Milk policy of 1970–71, a special analysis of the information obtained in the 1967–68 study was made to investigate any relationship between milk consumption and stature; the results were, however, inconclusive (Section 8). The wide variations in milk consumption were not explained by economic differences; dislikes and indispositions were recorded in many cases, but in others there was no apparent reason for the low intake.

10.5   Obesity

10.5.1 It was not practicable to include skinfold measurements in this study. In any case Quetelet's index may prove to be a more reliable index of any change in the prevalence of overweight in young children, because systematic inter-observer differences in measurement of height and weight are smaller than those of skinfold measurements (para 9.6).

10.5.2 A relationship is often suspected between the degree of overweight in an individual (child or adult) and the intake of carbohydrate or of "added sugars" in the food. The individual case records of those children in each age group with the 10% highest Quetelet's index were scrutinized, but few of these appeared also among the 10% of children who, in any age group, had the highest intake of either carbohydrate or "added sugars". This does not, however, refute the hypothesis that an excess of sucrose in the diet, which causes energy intake to be greater than energy output, is associated with the development of obesity. Once obesity is established, a child may become much less active and may decrease his or her energy intake.

10.6　Children from families with low incomes

10.6.1 Most of the children in the poor households described in paras 9.4.1–9.4.5 were on diets no lower in nutritional content than were the rest of the survey sample. Seven ate diets which were low in energy, and their intakes may or may not have been limited for financial reasons. If this were so, it is surprising that the nutritional quality, as opposed to the quantity, of their diet did not deteriorate. There may have been aspects of their environment unrevealed by the survey which restricted their activity, and so their requirement, and therefore their consumption, of food.

10.6.2 There were three children whose nutrient intakes were below an arbitrary level of 80% of the average for their age group (para 9.4.3), and these children were below average in height although not in weight. Their records did not provide any clear reason for low nutrient intakes. It needs to be remembered that even though others in the group of poorer families may have managed well enough, a great deal depends on the intelligence and capability of the mother or home-maker. (The changes in arrangements for Welfare milk that were announced in October 1970 contained specific provisions designed to safeguard the supply of free milk to poorer families.)

11. Summary of findings

11.1   The sample of children studied in each family size group was nationally representative of Great Britain: the 2 321 pre-school children were selected from 39 areas in England, Scotland and Wales (para 2.2.1). For various reasons, 236 of these children were found to be outside the scope of the survey (para 4.1) and an interview could not be obtained from 147 others (para 4.2). Thus the effective sample was 1 938 children, and although full dietary information was obtained on only two-thirds of them, something is known about nearly all the children (Section 4, paras 7.1.1–7.1.3 and 10.1.1–10.1.4).

11.2   In the analysis of results, subjects were grouped into four age groups, (1) 6 months and under 18 months; (2) $1\frac{1}{2}$ and under $2\frac{1}{2}$ years; (3) $2\frac{1}{2}$ and under $3\frac{1}{2}$ years; and (4) $3\frac{1}{2}$ and under $4\frac{1}{2}$ years (para 3.4.1). Most results refer to age/sex groups of children, but individual records have been scrutinized in special cases (Section 9).

11.3   The range of individual intakes of different foods and food groups and therefore of nutrients was very wide. This is to be expected since, on average, the bigger the child the more food he will need, and there will be variations in intake associated with differences in dietary pattern and with being "off-colour" (paras 10.2.1 and 10.2.2).

11.4   There was little difference in dietary pattern between children from families of different size.

11.5   Although milk was the most important source of nutrients to the youngest children, the dietary pattern included most of the foods in the mixed diet of an adult by eighteen months of age if not earlier (Diagrams A1–12, pp 68–79).

11.6   The average intakes of most nutrients reached or exceeded the levels recommended for all the age/sex groups of children (Department of Health and Social Security, 1969). The exceptions were vitamin D and iron (paras 6.3.5 and 6.4.1). Low dietary intakes of vitamin D are not necessarily of nutritional significance since this vitamin is obtained also by the action of sunlight on the skin. The intakes of iron reached the recommended levels in some but not all age/sex groups, but compared with the pilot study made in 1963 when a special study had failed to detect anaemia in these age groups, the 1967–68 study showed a larger intake of meat and this food is known to be a source from which dietary iron is particularly well absorbed (paras 10.2.3 and 10.2.4).

11.7   Groups of children from small families (Tables A7–10, pp 41–44), those in social classes I and II and III Non-Manual (Table A12, p 46), and those with the higher income levels (Table A14, p 48) derived a higher percentage of their energy intake from protein, although the recommended percentage was attained in all groups of children (paras 6.3.7 and 6.3.8).

11.8 The average daily energy intake of two-thirds (64%) of the children was below the recommended daily intake for their age, whereas by definition (Department of Health and Social Security, 1969) about 50% of children might have been expected to have intakes below those recommended for the age groups in this study. However, since the social and economic gradients of energy intake were in the opposite direction to what would have been expected had the children been undernourished, it is possible that the recommended daily intake of energy for these ages has been set too high (paras 6.3.4 and 10.3.1).

11.9 Groups of children from larger families and in social classes IV and V had higher average daily intakes of energy than the others, which is the opposite of what one would expect were the children undernourished (paras 6.3.6, 6.3.7 and 10.3.1; Tables A12 and 14, pp 46 and 48). These children did not weigh more than the others (para 7.5.3), and the difference in intakes could be due to a difference in energy requirement if, as seems possible, children with more siblings and with fewer social amenities were physically more active (para 10.3.2).

11.10 The mean daily intakes of energy, carbohydrate and "added sugars" were lower (the two last to a statistically significant extent), and those of all other nutrients higher, in children whose mothers stayed at school after the age of 15 years. Differences in intake where the mother was in paid employment were not so marked (para 6.3.9).

11.11 Heights and weights were adjusted for age, and the means and the standard deviations in age and sex groups were determined (para 7.3).

11.12 In older children there is known to be a social class/family size gradient in height, children from smaller families and social classes I and II being on average taller than the others. In this survey although height tended to be lower in the larger families, and to be related to social class, statistically significant relationships were found only in some age/sex groups. This may have been due to the relatively small numbers within the different groups. Similarly the expected relationship between height and other environmental factors, for example, the income of the head of the household—children in higher income families usually being taller—was not demonstrated in the survey (paras 7.4.1 and 10.4.2).

11.13 Although the average intakes of some nutrients (including protein) of groups of children from large families and social classes IV and V were higher than those for children from small families and social classes I and II (paras 6.3.6 and 6.3.7), there was no evidence that these differences were associated with any consistent or appreciable difference in height (para 7.5.2).

11.14 There was some evidence of a direct relationship between energy intake and height (para 7.5.2).

11.15 The possible relationship between milk intake and height noted in the 1963 pilot survey (para 8.4) was not immediately established in this survey.

34

Although in most groups there was a tendency for height to increase with milk intake, it was only slight and not consistent. A simple regression analysis revealed a significant relationship (P = 0.05) between height and milk intake only for boys aged $1\frac{1}{2}$ and under $2\frac{1}{2}$ years (paras 8.5 and 8.6).

11.16   A few children drank very little milk, much less than the average for their age. They were from families of all sizes and social classes, and in general were neither shorter nor lighter than the mean for their age group (paras 9.1.1 and 9.1.2).

11.17   There was little evidence in this survey that those groups of children who ate the most "added sugars" were overweight (paras 9.2.1–9.2.4) but the number of children considered in this analysis was small. They came pre-dominantly from large families of social classes III Manual, IV and V, and it is suggested that such children may be more active physically. Allowing for the difference in age of the groups, the average intake of "added sugars" by all groups of children was greater in this survey than in the pilot study of 1963 (para 6.4.1 and Table A16, p 50).

11.18   The study did not include skin-fold measurements, and Quetelet's index (footnote, p 21) was used as an index of overweight. Children with the 10% highest Quetelet's index were not characteristically predominant among the 10% of children who ate most "added sugar" or carbohydrate (paras 9.6. 10.5.1 and 10.5.2).

11.19   Children from families with low incomes were under-represented among those who produced usable diet records (para 5.3.2), but most of these children ate diets which were no worse than the rest of the survey sample (para 10.6.1.) Three of the 31 children from these families had an intake of all nutrients less than 80% (an arbitrarily selected level) of the mean intake for children of the same age and sex. These three children were shorter than the average for their age but were not below average weight (paras 9.4.1–9.4.5 and 10.6.2).

11.20   Among the 10% of children with the lowest energy intake for each age/ sex group, all family sizes, social classes and income groups were represented, and the quality of the diet did not differ significantly from that of all the survey children of the same age and sex. About half these children were said by the mother to have been unwell during the week of the survey. In each age/sex group, the average height of these children was less than 1% different from that of the other 90% of the children (either shorter or taller). The difference in average weight was 3–8% less than the weight of the other 90% of children (paras 9.3.1–9.3.5).

11.21   Dental studies

There was no very impressive relationship between the use of reservoir feeders and incisor caries; the relationship between dental caries and various factors was studied and is reported on by a senior dental officer of the Department in Appendix E (p 118).

12. References

Bransby, E. R. and Fothergill, J. E., 1954.
The diets of young children.
British Journal of Nutrition, **8**, 195–204.

Davie, R., Butler, N. and Goldstein, H., 1972.
From birth to seven: the second report of the National Child Development Study (1958 Cohort), with full statistical appendix.
Longman, in association with the National Children's Bureau, 1972.

Department of Health and Social Security, 1969.
Recommended intakes of nutrients for the United Kingdom.
Reports on Public Health and Medical Subjects, No. 120, London, H.M.S.O.

Department of Health and Social Security, 1971.
A nutrition survey of pregnant women 1967–68.
Unpublished but available to *bona fide* research workers.

Department of Health and Social Security, 1972.
A nutrition survey of the elderly.
Reports on Health and Social Subjects, No. 3, London, H.M.S.O.

Heimendinger, J., 1964.
Die Ergebnisse von Körpermessungen an 5000 Basler Kindern von 2–18 Jahren.
Helvetica Paediatrica Acta, **19**, Suppl. 13, 1–131.

Kemsley, W. F. F., Billewicz, W. Z. and Thomson, A. M., 1962.
A new weight-for-height standard based on British anthropometric data.
British Journal of Preventive and Social Medicine, **16**, 189–195.

Ministry of Agriculture, Fisheries and Food, 1969 and 1970.
Household food consumption and expenditure: 1967 and 1968.
Reports of the National Food Survey Committee, London, H.M.S.O.

Ministry of Health, 1968.
A pilot survey of the nutrition of young children in 1963.
Reports on Public Health and Medical Subjects, No. 118, London, H.M.S.O.

Paul, A. A., 1969.
The calculation of nicotinic acid equivalents and retinol equivalents in the British diet.
Nutrition, **23**, 131–136.

Scottish Home and Health Department, 1972.
Personal communication.

Tanner, J. M., Whitehouse, R. H. and Takaishi, M., 1966.
Standards from birth to maturity for height, weight, height velocity and weight velocity: British children, 1965.
Archives of Disease in Childhood, **41**, 454–471; 613–635.

Weiner, J. S. and Lourie, J. A., 1969.
Human biology: guide to field methods.
IBP Handbook, No. 9, p. 8. Oxford, Blackwell Scientific.

13. Appendix A
Detailed Tables and Diagrams

For a list, see pp xiii-xvi

Table A1: *The number of diet records obtained from children of different age groups in families of different sizes*[1]

Age group (years)	All family sizes	1 or 2 children	3 children	4 or more children
6 months and under 18 months	201	94	57	50
$1\frac{1}{2}$ and under $2\frac{1}{2}$	394	155	135	104
$2\frac{1}{2}$ and under $3\frac{1}{2}$	407	147	145	115
$3\frac{1}{2}$ and under $4\frac{1}{2}$	319	110	119	90
All age groups (a)	1321	506	456	359
Number interviewed (b) who were within the scope of the survey	1938	678	656	604
Percentage (a) of (b)	68.2	74.6	69.5	59.4

[1]Children under 15 years of age.

Table A2: *The number of dental and medical examinations of children in different age groups and in families of different sizes*[1]

Age group (years)	All family sizes	1 or 2 children	3 children	4 or more children
Dental examinations				
All ages	738	281	268	189
$1\frac{1}{2}$ and under $2\frac{1}{2}$	270	110	94	66
$2\frac{1}{2}$ and under $3\frac{1}{2}$	259	97	92	70
$3\frac{1}{2}$ and under $4\frac{1}{2}$	209	74	82	53
Medical examinations				
All ages	89	31	27	31
$1\frac{1}{2}$ and under $2\frac{1}{2}$	31	11	9	11
$2\frac{1}{2}$ and under $3\frac{1}{2}$	36	11	13	12
$3\frac{1}{2}$ and under $4\frac{1}{2}$	22	9	5	8

[1]Children under 15 years of age.

Table A3: *The number of diet records obtained in each quarter of the year from children in different age groups and in families of different sizes[1]*

Age group (years)	All family sizes	1 or 2 children	3 children	4 or more children
October—December 1967				
All ages	325	130	105	90
6 months and under 18 months	70	30	23	17
1½ and under 2½	82	35	26	21
2½ and under 3½	102	41	35	26
3½ and under 4½	71	24	21	26
January—March 1968				
All ages	349	140	119	90
6 months and under 18 months	63	33	17	13
1½ and under 2½	116	46	41	29
2½ and under 3½	94	31	31	32
3½ and under 4½	76	30	30	16
April—June 1968				
All ages	317	119	109	89
6 months and under 18 months	40	18	13	9
1½ and under 2½	95	40	31	24
2½ and under 3½	97	34	34	29
3½ and under 4½	85	27	31	27
July—September 1968				
All ages	330	117	123	90
6 months and under 18 months	28	13	4	11
1½ and under 2½	101	34	37	30
2½ and under 3½	114	41	45	28
3½ and under 4½	87	29	37	21

[1]Children under 15 years of age.

Table A4: *The number of children for whom diet records were and were not obtained from households of different family sizes[1] and different social classes*

Social class	All family sizes No.	%	1 or 2 children No.	%	3 children No.	%	4 or more children No.	%
Respondents who produced diet records								
I and II	238	18	95	19	86	19	57	16
III Non-Manual	121	9	60	12	41	9	20	6
III Manual	638	48	246	48	223	49	169	47
IV and V	287	22	90	18	95	21	102	28
Others[2]	37	3	15	3	11	2	11	3
Other respondents								
I and II	69	12	32	20	22	12	15	7
III Non-Manual	31	6	10	6	8	5	13	6
III Manual	276	49	73	45	93	51	110	51
IV and V	165	30	42	26	53	29	70	32
Others[2]	19	3	5	3	6	3	8	4

[1]Children under 15 years of age.

[2]Including armed forces, and unclassified because insufficient or no information was available.

Table A5: *The number of children for whom diet records were, and were not obtained from households of different family sizes[1] and different income groups according to the income of the head of the household*

Income group	All family sizes		1 or 2 children		3 children		4 or more children	
	No.	%	No.	%	No.	%	No.	%
Respondents who produced diet records								
£32 or more	128	10	47	9	53	11	28	8
£19 but less than £32	647	49	266	53	205	45	176	49
£11 but less than £19	515	39	176	35	190	42	149	41
Under £11	31	2	17	3	8	2	6	2
Other respondents								
£32 or more	40	7	15	9	15	8	10	5
£19 but less than £32	222	40	69	43	70	39	83	38
£11 but less than £19	275	49	70	43	90	49	115	53
Under £11	23	4	8	5	7	4	8	4

[1]Children under 15 years of age.

Table A6: *The percentage of households[1] who participated in the National Food Survey 1967 and 1968 in different income groups according to the income of the head of the household*

1967		1968	
Income group	%	Income group	%
£32 or more	11.8	£33 or more	13.6
£19 but less than £32	37.7	£19 but less than £33	44.3
£11 but less than £19	42.2	£11 10s but less than £19	34.0
Under £11:		Under £11 10s:	
Households with earners	4.7	Households with earners	4.9
Households without earners	3.6	Households without earners	3.2

[1]All households, except those solely or mainly dependent on old age pensions.

SOURCE: Ministry of Agriculture, Fisheries and Food (1969 and 1970).

Table A7: *Mean daily intake of energy and nutrients, and standard errors of the mean, of children from families of different sizes (numbers of children in parentheses)*
Age group 1: ½ and under 1½ yr.

Nutrient		1 or 2 children in family (94)		3 children in family (57)		4 or more children in family (50)	
		Mean	S.E.	Mean	S.E.	Mean	S.E.
Energy	kcal	1036	25	1045	35	1084	37
	MJ	4.3		4.4		4.5	
Animal protein	g	24.9	0.8	26.0	1.1	23.2	1.1
Total protein	g	33.8	0.9	34.5	1.3	33.3	1.2
Fat	g	42	1.3	43	1.9	44	1.9
Total carbohydrate	g	139	3.8	138	4.7	148	5.6
"Added sugars"[1]	g	45.9	2.1	48.0	3.2	51.9	3.1
Calcium	mg	770	23	790	36	740	32
Iron	mg	7.9	0.42	7.6	0.59	7.1	0.43
Vitamin A	iu	3260	234	2570	252	2050	137
	µg	980		770		620	
Thiamin	mg	0.7	0.05	0.6	0.07	0.6	0.03
Riboflavin	mg	1.3	0.09	1.4	0.13	1.1	0.04
Nicotinic acid	mg	6.7	0.92	6.5	1.19	5.4	0.31
Vitamin C	mg	51	3.5	42	3.3	44	4.5
Vitamin D	iu	261	25.1	193	27.1	154	17.2
	µg	6.5		4.8		3.9	
Pyridoxine	mg	0.6	0.05	0.6	0.07	0.5	0.02
Mean % energy derived from:—							
Total protein		13.2	0.2	13.3	0.3	12.4	0.3
Fat		36.2	0.6	36.4	0.7	36.0	0.8
"Added sugars"[1]		17.9	0.8	18.6	1.2	19.3	1.1
Other carbohydrate		32.7	NA	31.7	NA	32.3	NA

[1]For definition see paragraph 3.2.3.
NA = not applicable.

41

Table A8: Mean daily intake of energy and nutrients, and standard errors of the mean, of children from families of different sizes (numbers of children in parentheses)
Age group 2: 1½ and under 2½ yr.

Nutrient		1 or 2 children in family (155)		3 children in family (135)		4 or more children in family (104)	
		Mean	S.E.	Mean	S.E.	Mean	S.E.
Energy	kcal	1226	24	1266	28	1308	34
	MJ	5.1		5.3		5.5	
Animal protein	g	27.9	0.7	26.6	0.8	26.4	0.9
Total protein	g	38.2	0.8	37.6	1.0	38.4	1.1
Fat	g	54	1.2	54	1.5	55	1.7
Total carbohydrate	g	156	3.4	166	3.8	174	4.7
"Added sugars"[1]	g	53.9	1.7	58.5	2.1	58.8	2.3
Calcium	mg	700	17.4	690	23.6	680	23.9
Iron	mg	6.5	0.20	6.7	0.27	6.5	0.23
Vitamin A	iu	2880	176	2320	160	2190	164
	µg	860		700		660	
Thiamin	mg	0.6	0.02	0.6	0.02	0.6	0.02
Riboflavin	mg	1.1	0.03	1.1	0.04	1.1	0.04
Nicotinic acid	mg	6.8	0.30	6.3	0.22	6.5	0.25
Vitamin C	mg	44	2.8	41	3.5	35	3.4
Vitamin D	iu	147	17.3	99	12.8	87	11.0
Pyridoxine	µg	3.7		2.5		2.2	
	mg	0.6	0.02	0.6	0.02	0.7	0.02
Mean % of calories derived from:—							
Total protein		12.5	0.1	11.9	0.1	11.8	0.2
Fat		39.5	0.4	38.5	0.4	37.7	0.5
"Added sugars"[1]		17.6	0.5	18.5	0.5	18.2	0.6
Other carbohydrate		30.4	NA	31.1	NA	32.3	NA

[1] For definition see paragraph 3.2.3.
NA = not applicable.

42

Table A9: *Mean daily intake of energy and nutrients, and standard errors of the mean, of children from families of different sizes (numbers of children in parentheses)*
Age group 3: 2½ and under 3½ yr.

Nutrient		1 or 2 children in family (147)		3 children in family (145)		4 or more children in family (115)	
		Mean	S.E.	Mean	S.E.	Mean	S.E.
Energy	kcal	1343	25	1406	30	1469	39
	MJ	5.6		5.9		6.1	
Animal protein	g	27.6	0.7	28.2	0.8	27.6	0.9
Total protein	g	39.5	0.8	40.8	1.0	42.0	1.2
Fat	g	58	1.2	60	1.6	61	1.9
Total carbohydrate	g	176	3.6	185	4.0	199	5.7
"Added sugars"[1]	g	63.3	1.9	65.2	2.0	66.0	2.5
Calcium	mg	640	15.7	670	18.0	670	22.0
Iron	mg	6.5	0.17	6.7	0.17	7.2	0.33
Vitamin A	iu	2390	140	2070	106	2210	217
	µg	720		620		660	
Thiamin	mg	0.7	0.02	0.7	0.02	0.7	0.02
Riboflavin	mg	1.0	0.03	1.1	0.03	1.1	0.04
Nicotinic acid	mg	7.1	0.25	7.2	0.24	7.8	0.31
Vitamin C	mg	40	2.9	39	2.9	30	1.9
Vitamin D	iu	88	9.4	64	5.4	92	12.9
	µg	2.2		1.6		2.3	
Pyridoxine	mg	0.7	0.02	0.7	0.02	0.7	0.02
Mean % of calories derived from:—							
Total protein		11.8	0.1	11.6	0.1	11.5	0.2
Fat		38.7	0.4	38.3	0.3	37.3	0.5
"Added sugars"[1]		18.9	0.5	18.7	0.5	18.1	0.5
Other carbohydrate		30.6	NA	31.4	NA	33.1	NA

[1]For definition see paragraph 3.2.3
NA = not applicable.

43

Table A10: Mean daily intake of energy and nutrients, and standard errors of the mean, of children from families of different sizes (numbers of children in parentheses)
Age group: 4: 3½ and under 4½ yr.

Nutrient		1 or 2 children in family (110)		3 children in family (119)		4 or more children in family (90)	
		Mean	S.E.	Mean	S.E.	Mean	S.E.
Energy	kcal	1422	33	1439	33	1564	46
	MJ	6.0		6.0		6.5	
Animal protein	g	28.3	0.9	26.7	0.8	28.0	1.0
Total protein	g	41.0	1.1	40.6	1.0	43.8	1.4
Fat	g	61	1.8	60	1.8	66	2.4
Total carbohydrate	g	189	4.4	195	4.2	211	5.8
"Added sugars"[1]	g	69.2	2.1	68.2	2.1	71.0	2.7
Calcium	mg	670	20.6	630	16.8	700	26.9
Iron	mg	6.9	0.21	6.9	0.20	7.5	0.24
Vitamin A	iu	2500	193	2260	150	2440	188
	μg	750		680		730	
Thiamin	mg	0.7	0.03	0.7	0.02	0.8	0.03
Riboflavin	mg	1.1	0.03	1.0	0.03	1.1	0.05
Nicotinic acid	mg	7.9	0.33	7.4	0.23	8.5	0.39
Vitamin C	mg	45	4.0	35	2.4	32	2.3
Vitamin D	iu	73	8.5	66	9.3	81	10.5
	μg	1.8		1.7		2.0	
Pyridoxine	mg	0.7	0.02	0.7	0.02	0.8	0.03
Mean % of energy derived from:—							
Total protein		11.5	0.1	11.3	0.1	11.2	0.2
Fat		38.0	0.5	37.5	0.4	37.4	0.4
"Added sugars"[1]		19.7	0.5	19.1	0.5	18.5	0.6
Other carbohydrate		30.8	NA	32.1	NA	32.9	NA

[1]For definition see paragraph 3.2.3.
NA = not applicable.

Table A11: *Recommended daily intakes of energy and nutrients for boys and girls in the United Kingdom*

Age range (years)	Body weight kg	Energy kcal	Energy MJ	Protein g	Thiamin mg	Riboflavin mg	Ascorbic acid mg	Vitamin A μg retinol equivalents	Vitamin D μg cholecal- ciferol	Calcium mg	Iron mg
0 up to 1	7.3	800	3.3	20	0.3	0.4	15	450	10	600[1]	6[1]
1 up to 2	11.4	1200	5.0	30	0.5	0.6	20	300	10	500	7
2 up to 3	13.5	1400	5.9	35	0.6	0.7	20	300	10	500	7
3 up to 5	16.5	1600	6.7	40	0.6	0.8	20	300	10	500	8

[1]These figures apply to infants who are not breast fed. Infants who are entirely breast fed receive smaller quantities; these are adequate since absorption from breast milk is higher.

NOTE: The recommended intake for nicotinic acid equivalents has been omitted because sufficient information about the tryptophan content of foods is not yet available to allow the dietary content of nicotinic acid to be expressed in mg of nicotinic acid equivalents.

SOURCE: Department of Health and Social Security (1969).

Table A12: *Mean daily intake of energy and nutrients of children from different social classes (number of children in parentheses)*

Nutrient		Social class				
		I & II (238)	III Non-Manual (121)	III Manual (638)	IV & V (287)	Others (37)
Energy	kcal	1286	1249	1325	1379	1314
	MJ	5.4	5.2	5.5	5.8	5.5
Animal protein	g	27.7	26.6	26.9	27.4	26.3
Total protein	g	38.7	37.5	39.0	40.2	39.0
Fat	g	56	53	56	58	55
Total carbohydrate	g	166	164	177	185	176
"Added sugars"[1]	g	57.5	57.9	61.9	63.5	57.0
Calcium	mg	680	700	680	700	680
Iron	mg	6.81	6.45	6.90	7.21	7.13
Vitamin A	iu	2740	2550	2400	2240	2110
	µg	820	770	720	670	630
Thiamin	mg	0.7	0.6	0.7	0.7	0.6
Riboflavin	mg	1.2	1.1	1.1	1.1	1.1
Nicotinic acid	mg	7.2	6.2	7.2	7.2	6.1
Vitamin C	mg	53	42	38	32	38
Vitamin D	iu	121	110	105	112	78
	µg	3.0	2.8	2.6	2.8	2.0
Pyridoxine	mg	0.7	0.6	0.7	0.7	0.7
Mean % energy derived from:						
Total protein		12.2	12.2	11.9	11.8	11.9
Fat		39.0	38.3	37.7	37.5	37.1
"Added sugars"[1]		17.9	18.7	18.8	18.5	18.3
Other carbohydrate		30.9	30.8	31.6	32.2	32.7

[1]For definition see paragraph 3.2.3.

Table A 13: *Mean daily intake of vitamin C (mg) of children from families of different sizes and different social classes (standard errors of the mean in parentheses)*

Size of family	Intake	All social classes	Social class I and II	Social class III Non-Manual	Social class III Manual	Social class IV and V	Others
All	Mean	40 (0.9)	53 (2.8)	42 (3.3)	38 (1.3)	32 (1.4)	38 (3.9)
	Number of children	1321	238	121	638	287	37
1 or 2 children	Mean	44 (1.6)	57 (4.6)	47 (5.2)	42 (2.2)	36 (2.8)	42 (6.2)
	Number of children	506	95	60	246	90	15
3 children	Mean	39 (1.6)	56 (5.2)	40 (5.6)	35 (1.8)	32 (2.4)	37 (8.9)
	Number of children	456	86	41	223	95	11
4 or more children	Mean	34 (1.5)	41 (4.1)	30 (4.1)	35 (2.5)	29 (1.9)	33 (5.1)
	Number of children	359	57	20	169	102	11

47

Table A14: *Mean daily intake of energy and nutrients of children in relation to the income of the head of the household (number of children in parentheses)*

Nutrient		Weekly income of head of household			
		Under £11	£11 but less than £19	£19 but less than £32	£32 or more
		(31)	(515)	(647)	(128)
Energy	kcal	1320	1338	1320	1269
	MJ	5.5	5.6	5.5	5.3
Animal protein	g	24.8	26.7	27.2	28.9
Total protein	g	37.3	39.1	39.1	39.6
Fat	g	54	56	56	57
Total carbohydrate	g	181	179	175	159
"Added sugars"[1]	g	63.3	61.5	61.7	53.9
Calcium	mg	600	700	680	690
Iron	mg	6.8	6.8	7.0	7.1
Vitamin A	iu	1850	2290	2470	2910
	µg	560	690	740	870
Thiamin	mg	0.6	0.7	0.7	0.7
Riboflavin	mg	0.9	1.1	1.1	1.2
Nicotinic acid	mg	6.3	7.0	7.0	7.7
Vitamin C	mg	38	34	41	57
Vitamin D	iu	78	109	107	129
	µg	2.0	2.7	2.7	3.2
Pyridoxine	mg	0.7	0.7	0.7	0.8
Mean % energy derived from:					
Total protein		11.4	11.8	11.9	12.6
Fat		36.9	37.6	37.8	39.9
"Added sugars"[1]		19.4	18.5	18.8	17.2

[1]For definition see paragraph 3.2.3.

Table A15: *Mean daily intake of energy and nutrients of children in relation to the age at which the mother left school and whether or not she was working (number of children in parentheses)*

Nutrient		Age at which mother left school		Mother working	Mother not working
		15 and under (999)	16 and over (321)	(166)	(1155)
Energy	kcal	1329	1296	1383	1314
	MJ	5.6	5.4	5.8	5.5
Animal protein	g	26.7	28.2	28.2	26.9
Total protein	g	38.9	39.5	40.9	38.8
Fat	g	56	56	60	56
Total carbohydrate	g	177	168	181	174
"Added sugars"[1]	g	61.7	58.5	61.9	60.8
Calcium	mg	680	690	690	690
Iron	mg	6.9	7.1	6.9	6.9
Vitamin A	iu	2290	2880	2330	2450
	µg	690	860	700	740
Thiamin	mg	0.6	0.7	0.7	0.7
Riboflavin	mg	1.1	1.2	1.1	1.1
Nicotinic acid	mg	7.0	7.4	7.3	7.0
Vitamin C	mg	36	51	36	40
Vitamin D	iu	102	134	94	112
	µg	2.6	3.4	2.4	2.8
Pyridoxine	mg	0.7	0.7	0.7	0.7
Mean % energy derived from:					
Total protein		11.8	12.3	11.9	11.9
Fat		37.7	38.6	38.6	37.8
"Added sugars"[1]		18.7	18.2	18.0	18.6

[1] For definition see paragraph 3.2.3.

49

Table A16: *Mean daily intake of energy and nutrients of children in surveys of 1951 (Bransby and Fothergill, 1954), 1963 (Ministry of Health, 1968) and 1967–68 (this survey)*

Nutrient		1951 B and F 6–12 months	1963 MOH 9–12 months	1967–68 this survey¹ 6–18 months	1951 B and F 1–2 years	1963 MOH 1–2 years	1967–68 this survey¹ 1½–2½ years	1951 B and F 2–3 years	1963 MOH 2–3 years	1967–68 this survey¹ 2½–3½ years	1951 B and F 3–4 years	1963 MOH 3–4 years	1967–68 this survey¹ 3½–4½ years	1951 B and F 4–5 years	1963 MOH 4–5 years
Energy	kcal	1080	980	1050	1330	1117	1262	1540	1349	1401	1590	1341	1468	1730	1545
	MJ	4.5	4.1	4.4	5.6	4.7	5.3	6.4	5.6	5.9	6.7	5.6	6.1	7.2	6.5
Animal protein	g	28	24.5	24.8	25	25.7	27.1	27	28.8	27.8	27	27.2	27.6	28	30.1
Total protein	g	38	32.2	33.9	41	34.5	38.0	46	40.3	40.7	47	39.1	41.6	51	44.3
Fat	g	46	42	42.6	59	51	54.4	69	61	59.7	70	58	61.9	76	68
Total carbohydrate	g	131	125	141	160	137	164	185	170	186	194	176	197	214	201
Calcium	mg	970	838	771	750	708	691	720	696	658	730	641	661	760	697
Iron	mg	6.7	8.0	7.6	7.8	7.2	6.6	8.3	7.1	6.8	8.3	6.4	7.1	9.0	7.5
Vitamin A	iu	2160	2031	2762	2340	2125	2505	2290	2505	2224	2320	2313	2391	2380	2655
	µg	650	610	830	700	640	750	690	750	670	700	690	720	710	800
Thiamin	mg	0.58	0.62	0.64	0.65	0.63	0.62	0.69	0.64	0.67	0.70	0.63	0.70	0.77	0.72
Riboflavin	mg	1.18	1.23	1.25	0.99	1.09	1.07	1.02	1.13	1.07	1.01	1.08	1.08	1.03	1.19
Nicotinic acid	mg	2.7	4.4	6.3	4.4	5.4	6.5	5.4	6.0	7.3	5.8	6.2	7.9	6.6	7.1
Vitamin C	mg	14	20	47	21	25	40	24	29	37	26	29	38	28	36
Vitamin D	iu	NA	222	215	NA	134	115	NA	110	81	NA	88	73	NA	98
	µg	NA	5.6	5.4	NA	3.4	2.9	NA	2.8	2.0	NA	2.2	1.8	NA	2.5
Pyridoxine	mg	NA	0.51	0.59	NA	0.56	0.65	NA	0.65	0.71	NA	0.65	0.73	NA	0.74
"Added sugars"²	g	NA	34	48	NA	43	57	NA	57	65	NA	60	69	NA	68

¹The different age groupings in the 1967–68 survey should be taken into account when making comparisons between the three surveys. The 1967–68 figures include the intakes from some supplements which are not included in figures from the two earlier surveys.

²For definition see paragraph 3.2.3.

NA—Not available.

Table A17: *Percentage distribution of boys in the survey aged 6 months and under $1\frac{1}{2}$ years according to height (adjusted for age) by family size[1], social class, income of head of household and age at which mother left school*

BOYS $\frac{1}{2}$ and under $1\frac{1}{2}$ years	Number of children	Height adjusted for age (cm)				
		up to 72.4 %	72.5– 74.9 %	75.0– 77.4 %	77.5– 79.9 %	80.0 and over %
Family size[1]						
1 or 2	52	15	23	29	18	15
3	30	10	17	43	13	17
4 or more	21	24	24	9	24	19
Social class						
I and II	15	33	13	47	0	7
III Non-Manual	19	0	32	32	21	15
III Manual	47	23	21	26	15	15
IV and V	20	0	20	25	30	25
Income group						
£32 or more	13	31	15	38	8	8
£19 but under £32	47	17	21	36	13	13
£11 but under £19	42	10	24	19	26	21
under £11	1	0	0	0	0	100
School-leaving age of mother						
15 and under	69	13	22	25	23	17
over 15	34	21	21	38	6	14

[1]Number of children under 15 years of age.

Table A18: *Percentage distribution of boys in the survey aged $1\frac{1}{2}$–$2\frac{1}{2}$ years according to height (adjusted for age) by family size[1], social class, income of head of household and age at which mother left school*

BOYS $1\frac{1}{2}$ and under $2\frac{1}{2}$ years	Number of children	Height adjusted for age (cm)				
		up to 79.9 %	80.0– 82.4 %	82.5– 84.9 %	85.0– 87.4 %	87.5– 89.9 %	90.0 and over %
Family size[1]							
1 or 2	57	12	9	16	23	26	14
3	68	4	9	19	24	26	18
4 or more	61	6	5	20	39	15	15
Social class							
I and II	21	5	5	19	28	33	10
III Non-Manual	11	9	0	9	37	18	27
III Manual	102	9	10	18	27	18	18
IV and V	48	6	4	23	27	27	13
Income group							
£32 or more	11	0	0	18	37	27	18
£19 but under £32	96	9	6	17	27	24	17
£11 but under £19	76	7	9	21	29	20	14
under £11	3	0	33	0	33	34	0
School-leaving age of mother							
15 and under	147	7	7	21	27	21	17
over 15	39	8	8	10	36	28	10

[1]Number of children under 15 years of age.

Table A19: *Percentage distribution of boys in the survey aged 2½—3½ years according to height (adjusted for age) by family size[1], social class, income of head of household and age at which mother left school*

BOYS 2½ and under 3½ years	Number of children	Height adjusted for age (cm)						
		Up to 87.4 %	87.5– 89.9 %	90.0– 92.4 %	92.5– 94.9 %	95.0– 97.4 %	97.5– 99.9 %	100.0 and over %
Family size[1]								
1 or 2	73	4	6	16	23	25	18	8
3	69	7	6	10	23	18	23	18
4 or more	46	9	13	20	20	17	15	6
Social class								
I and II	39	8	5	13	26	15	23	10
III Non-Manual	19	0	16	5	21	26	32	0
III Manual	79	4	5	19	22	24	15	11
IV and V	47	13	11	13	23	15	17	8
Income group								
£32 or more	20	5	10	25	30	10	15	5
£19 but under £32	98	4	6	13	22	24	20	11
£11 but under £19	68	10	9	15	20	18	19	9
under £11	2	0	0	0	50	50	0	0
School-leaving age of mother								
15 and under	137	7	8	15	21	20	20	9
over 15	50	4	6	16	26	20	18	10

[1]Number of children under 15 years of age.

Table A20: *Percentage distribution of boys in the survey aged 3½—4½ years according to height (adjusted for age) by family size[1], social class, income of head of household and age at which mother left school*

BOYS 3½ and under 4½ years	Number of children	Height adjusted for age (cm)						
		Up to 94.9 %	95.0– 97.4 %	97.5– 99.9 %	100.0– 102.4 %	102.5– 104.9 %	105.0– 107.4 %	107.5 and over %
Family size[1]								
1 or 2	54	7	9	17	26	13	13	15
3	66	8	10	12	33	15	14	8
4 or more	44	2	11	18	23	18	21	7
Social class								
I and II	29	7	4	7	31	31	10	10
III Non-Manual	16	6	12	25	19	6	19	13
III Manual	89	6	11	17	30	11	15	10
IV and V	27	7	15	15	19	15	22	7
Income Group								
£32 or more	13	0	8	8	38	38	0	8
£19 but under £32	77	6	9	16	25	18	16	10
£11 but under £19	66	6	14	17	24	7	18	9
under £11	8	12	0	13	37	13	12	13
School-leaving age of mother								
15 and under	123	8	10	17	27	14	14	10
over 15	41	0	10	10	32	19	19	10

[1]Number of children under 15 years of age.

Table A21 : *Percentage distribution of girls in the survey aged 6 months–1½ years according to height (adjusted for age) by family size[1], social class, income of head of household and age at which mother left school*

GIRLS ½ and under 1½ years	Number of children	Height adjusted for age (cm)				
		Up to 69.9 %	70.0– 72.4 %	72.5– 74.9 %	75.0– 77.4 %	77.5 and over %
Family size[1]						
1 or 2	42	12	17	21	26	24
3	28	11	18	32	14	25
4 or more	26	23	19	35	19	4
Social class						
I and II	21	10	9	38	19	24
III Non-Manual	6	17	17	0	50	16
III Manual	44	11	23	27	16	23
IV and V	23	26	13	30	22	9
Income group						
£32 or more	11	9	9	46	18	18
£19 but under £32	53	11	21	28	23	17
£11 but under £19	32	22	15	22	19	22
under £11	0	0	0	0	0	0
School-leaving age of mother						
15 and under	74	16	20	24	22	18
over 15	22	9	9	41	18	23

[1]Number of children under 15 years of age.

Table A22 : *Percentage distribution of girls in the survey aged 1½–2½ years according to height (adjusted for age) by family size[1], social class, income of head of household and age at which mother left school*

GIRLS 1½ and under 2½ years	Number of children	Height adjusted for age (cm)				
		Up to 79.9 %	80.0– 82.4 %	82.5– 84.9 %	85.0– 87.4 %	87.5– 89.9 %	90.0 and over %
Family size[1]						
1 or 2	81	4	11	19	41	18	7
3	57	9	18	19	28	19	7
4 or more	43	14	14	30	21	9	12
Social class						
I and II	38	10	8	24	29	16	13
III Non-Manaual	14	7	14	21	29	29	0
III Manual	83	8	14	21	30	17	10
IV and V	38	5	16	24	39	13	3
Income group						
£32 or more	18	28	5	17	28	17	5
£19 but under £32	82	7	15	23	26	21	8
£11 but under £19	77	4	14	22	39	12	9
under £11	4	0	25	0	50	25	0
School-leaving age of mother						
15 and under	140	6	16	22	34	16	6
over 15	41	12	7	20	24	20	17

[1]Number of children under 15 years of age.

Table A23: *Percentage of girls in the survey aged $2\frac{1}{2}$–$3\frac{1}{2}$ years according to height (adjusted for age) by family size[1], social class, income of head of household and age at which mother left school*

GIRLS $2\frac{1}{2}$ and under $3\frac{1}{2}$ years	Number of children	Height adjusted for age (cm)					
		up to 87.4 %	87.5– 89.9 %	90.0– 92.4 %	92.5– 94.9 %	95.0– 97.4 %	97.5 and over %
Family size[1]							
1 or 2	69	4	6	25	23	29	13
3	69	7	12	16	28	20	17
4 or more	56	20	11	21	18	18	12
Social class							
I and II	44	9	11	14	30	16	20
III Non-Manual	16	13	0	25	31	31	0
III Manual	92	9	12	20	22	23	14
IV and V	35	11	3	26	17	29	14
Income group							
£32 or more	24	8	8	17	38	12	17
£19 but under £32	93	7	13	16	19	28	17
£11 but under £19	71	14	4	25	26	20	11
under £11	6	17	17	50	0	16	0
School-leaving age of mother							
15 and under	143	11	8	23	22	24	12
over 15	51	6	14	14	27	18	21

[1]Number of children under 15 years of age.

Table A24: *Percentage distribution of girls in the survey aged $3\frac{1}{2}$–$4\frac{1}{2}$ years according to height (adjusted for age) by family size[1], social class, income of head of household and age at which mother left school*

GIRLS $3\frac{1}{2}$ and under $4\frac{1}{2}$ years	Number of children	Height adjusted for age (cm)					
		up to 94.9 %	95.0– 97.4 %	97.5– 99.9 %	100.0– 102.4 %	102.5– 104.9 %	105.0 and over %
Family size[1]							
1 or 2	53	10	13	11	26	25	15
3	46	4	9	15	30	22	20
4 or more	43	21	9	26	28	7	9
Social class							
I and II	25	0	8	16	28	20	28
III Non-Manual	14	0	7	36	21	7	29
III Manual	66	15	11	13	30	20	11
IV and V	34	17	15	18	26	18	6
Income group							
£32 or more	15	0	7	33	20	13	27
£19 but under £32	67	12	11	13	24	22	18
£11 but under £19	56	14	13	16	36	12	9
under £11	4	0	0	25	25	50	0
School-leaving age of mother							
15 and under	110	14	11	16	25	18	16
over 15	32	3	9	19	38	19	12

[1]Number of children under 15 years of age.

Table A25: *Mean daily intake of energy and protein of children of different heights (adjusted for age) within the different age/sex groups*

Age group (years)	BOYS					GIRLS				
	Adjusted height cm	Number of children	Energy kcal MJ	Protein g	Protein per 1000 kcal	Adjusted height cm	Number of children	Energy kcal MJ	Protein g	Protein per 1000 kcal
½ and under 1½	All	103	1053 4.4	33.7	32.0	All	96	1049 4.4	34.5	32.9
	Under 75.0	38	1027 4.3	32.9	32.0	Under 72.5	31	1107 4.6	36.9	33.3
	75.0–77.4	30	1086 4.5	35.1	32.3	72.5–74.9	27	1048 4.4	33.9	32.4
	77.5 and over	35	1053 4.4	33.4	31.7	75.0 and over	38	1002 4.2	33.0	32.9
1½ and under 2½	All	186	1273 5.3	38.5	30.2	All	181	1237 5.2	37.0	29.9
	Under 85.0	62	1303 5.5	39.2	30.1	Under 85.0	78	1259 5.3	37.6	29.9
	85.0–87.4	53	1293 5.4	38.7	29.9	85.0–87.4	58	1186 5.0	34.7	29.3
	87.5 and over	71	1231 5.2	37.6	30.5	87.5 and over	45	1262 5.3	38.9	30.8
2½ and under 3½	All	188	1466 6.1	42.3	28.9	All	194	1326 5.6	38.7	29.2
	Under 92.5	54	1374 5.8	39.6	28.8	Under 92.5	77	1247 5.2	36.0	28.9
	92.5–97.4	80	1508 6.3	43.9	29.1	92.5–94.9	45	1336 5.6	39.5	29.6
	97.5 and over	54	1496 6.3	42.5	28.4	95.0 and over	72	1406 5.9	41.0	29.2
3½ and under 4½	All	164	1534 6.4	44.0	28.7	All	142	1404 5.9	39.7	28.3
	Under 100.0	52	1461 6.1	42.0	28.8	Under 100.0	55	1427 6.0	39.0	27.3
	100.0–104.9	71	1585 6.6	45.4	28.6	100.0–102.4	40	1396 5.8	41.0	29.4
	105.0 and over	41	1539 6.4	43.9	28.5	102.5 and over	47	1385 5.8	39.3	28.4

Table A26: Mean daily intake of energy and protein of children of different weights (adjusted for age) within the different age/sex groups

Age group (years)	BOYS						GIRLS					
	Adjusted weight kg	Number of children	Energy kcal	Energy MJ	Protein g	Protein per 1000 kcal	Adjusted weight kg	Number of children	Energy kcal	Energy MJ	Protein g	Protein per 1000 kcal
½ and under 1½	All	104	1063	4.5	34.0	32.0	All	99	1049	4.4	34.4	32.8
	Under 10 kg	28	1068	4.5	33.6	31.5	Under 9 kg	23	1006	4.2	33.1	32.9
	10 kg and under 11 kg	28	1003	4.2	31.7	31.6	9 kg and under 10 kg	31	996	4.2	32.2	32.3
	11 kg and over	48	1096	4.6	35.6	32.5	10 kg and over	45	1108	4.6	36.6	33.0
1½ and under 2½	All	200	1277	5.3	38.6	30.2	All	194	1235	5.2	37.1	30.0
	Under 12 kg	55	1209	5.1	35.7	29.5	Under 12 kg	84	1192	5.0	35.7	30.0
	12 kg and under 13 kg	62	1304	5.5	39.8	30.5	12 kg and under 13 kg	56	1255	5.3	36.7	29.2
	13 kg and over	83	1303	5.5	39.6	30.4	13 kg and over	54	1281	5.4	39.5	30.8
2½ and under 3½	All	195	1472	6.2	42.3	28.7	All	200	1335	5.6	39.0	29.2
	Under 14 kg	67	1420	5.9	40.4	28.5	Under 13 kg	55	1226	5.1	34.7	28.3
	14 kg and under 16 kg	88	1459	6.1	42.8	29.3	13 kg and under 15 kg	94	1345	5.6	39.5	29.4
	16 kg and over	40	1590	6.7	44.5	28.0	15 kg and over	51	1432	6.0	42.7	29.8
3½ and under 4½	All	167	1529	6.4	43.7	28.6	All	147	1409	5.9	39.8	28.3
	Under 16 kg	76	1435	6.0	40.8	28.4	Under 16 kg	75	1399	5.9	39.0	27.9
	16 kg and under 18 kg	55	1590	6.7	45.6	28.7	16 kg and under 17 kg	32	1364	5.7	38.9	28.5
	18 kg and over	36	1637	6.9	46.8	28.6	17 kg and over	40	1461	6.1	41.8	28.6

Table A27: *Mean daily intake of energy and protein related to Quetelet's index of children within the different age/sex groups*

Age group (years)	BOYS Quetelet's index[1]	Number of children	Energy kcal	Energy MJ	Protein g	Protein per 1000 kcal	GIRLS Quetelet's index[1]	Number of children	Energy kcal	Energy MJ	Protein g	Protein per 1000 kcal
½ and under 1½	All	102	1056	4.4	33.8	32.0	All	96	1048	4.4	34.5	32.9
	Under 1.80	40	1051	4.4	33.6	32.0	Under 1.70	28	993	4.2	31.9	32.1
	1.80–1.99	33	1049	4.4	33.4	31.8	1.70–1.89	39	996	4.2	33.4	33.5
	2.00 and over	29	1069	4.5	34.4	32.2	1.90 and over	29	1173	4.9	38.6	32.9
1½ and under 2½	All	186	1273	5.3	38.5	30.2	All	179	1235	5.2	37.0	30.0
	Under 1.60	36	1175	4.9	34.6	29.5	Under 1.60	60	1218	5.1	37.1	30.5
	1.60–1.79	81	1255	5.3	38.9	31.0	1.60–1.79	69	1250	5.2	36.0	28.8
	1.80 and over	69	1343	5.6	40.0	29.8	1.80 and over	50	1237	5.2	38.2	30.9
2½ and under 3½	All	186	1465	6.1	42.2	28.8	All	191	1327	5.6	38.7	29.2
	Under 1.60	69	1367	5.7	39.8	29.1	Under 1.50	42	1247	5.2	35.4	28.4
	1.60–1.69	52	1417	5.9	40.6	28.7	1.50–1.69	103	1344	5.6	38.8	28.9
	1.70 and over	65	1607	6.7	46.0	28.6	1.70 and over	46	1365	5.7	41.6	30.5
3½ and under 4½	All	163	1528	6.4	43.7	28.6	All	142	1404	5.9	39.7	28.3
	Under 1.50	34	1418	5.9	40.3	28.4	Under 1.50	38	1292	5.4	36.6	28.3
	1.50–1.69	94	1525	6.4	43.9	28.8	1.50–1.69	75	1439	6.0	40.0	27.8
	1.70 and over	35	1645	6.9	46.5	28.3	1.70 and over	29	1464	6.1	40.6	27.7

[1]Quetelet's index is $\dfrac{\text{weight (kg)}}{\text{height (cm)}^2} \times 1000.$

57

Table A28: *Contribution from milk to the mean daily intake of energy and some nutrients in children of different age groups (numbers of children in parentheses)*

Milk		Age group (years)			
		½ and under 1½ (201)	1½ and under 2½ (394)	2½ and under 3½ (407)	3½ and under 4½ (319)
Mean daily intake of milk (oz)		16.2	13.7	12.1	12.0
Range of intake		3.3–47.9	1.5–41.1	0.6–35.1	0.7–39.3
Contribution from milk of:					
Energy (kcal)	mean	308	260	230	228
	range	63–910	29–781	11–667	13–747
(MJ)	mean	1.3	1.1	1.0	1.0
	range	0.26–3.81	0.12–3.27	0.05–2.79	0.05–3.13
Total protein (g)	mean	14.6	12.3	10.9	10.8
	range	3.0–43.1	1.4–37.0	0.5–31.6	0.6–35.4
Calcium (mg)	mean	550	470	410	410
	range	110–1630	50–1400	20–1190	20–1340
Riboflavin (mg)	mean	0.6	0.5	0.5	0.5
	range	0.1–1.8	0.1–1.6	0.0–1.3	0.0–1.5
Contribution from milk as percentage of total intake:					
Energy	(%)	29	21	16	16
Total protein	(%)	43	32	27	26
Calcium	(%)	71	67	63	62
Riboflavin	(%)	49	49	43	42

Table A29: *Mean daily intake of energy and some nutrients of children aged ½ and under 1½ years from families of different sizes in 3 groups[1] according to the intake of milk (oz) from all sources*

Family size	Group	No. of children	Mean daily intake					
			Milk oz	Energy kcal	MJ	Total protein g	Calcium mg	Riboflavin mg
1–2 children	I	24	9.0	957	4.0	28.7	560	0.9
	II	45	15.2	1052	4.4	34.5	750	1.2
	III	25	24.4	1083	4.5	37.7	1020	1.8
3 children	I	14	9.6	896	3.7	28.6	510	0.8
	II	26	16.1	1047	4.4	34.2	750	1.5
	III	17	27.6	1164	4.9	39.9	1070	1.5
4 or more children	I	13	7.1	1082	4.5	29.8	490	0.8
	II	28	15.5	1057	4.4	32.6	760	1.1
	III	9	24.7	1171	4.9	40.4	1070	1.5

[1]Group I: below 25 percentile milk intake.
Group II: between 25th and 75th percentile milk intake.
Group III: above 75th percentile milk intake.

Table A30: *Mean daily intake of energy and some nutrients of children aged 1½ and under 2½ years from families of different sizes in 3 groups[1] according to the intake of milk (oz) from all sources*

Family size	Group	No. of children	Mean daily intake					
			Milk oz	Energy kcal	MJ	Total protein g	Calcium mg	Riboflavin mg
1–2 children	I	37	7.8	1145	4.8	32.4	480	0.8
	II	76	13.1	1193	5.0	37.5	670	1.1
	III	42	21.6	1359	5.7	44.5	940	1.4
3 children	I	35	7.9	1157	4.8	32.1	480	0.8
	II	70	13.3	1265	5.3	37.1	670	1.0
	III	30	23.1	1396	5.8	45.2	1000	1.5
4 or more children	I	27	7.3	1115	4.7	31.0	450	0.8
	II	50	12.7	1318	5.5	37.8	650	1.0
	III	27	21.5	1484	6.2	47.1	960	1.4

[1]Group I: below 25th percentile milk intake.
Group II: between 25th and 75th percentile milk intake.
Group III: above 75th percentile milk intake.

Table A31: *Mean daily intake of energy and some nutrients of children aged 2½ and under 3½ years from families of different sizes in 3 groups[1] according to the intake of milk (oz) from all sources*

Family size	Group	No. of children	Mean daily intake					
			Milk oz	Energy kcal	MJ	Total protein g	Calcium mg	Riboflavin mg
1–2 children	I	39	6.4	1174	4.9	32.9	430	0.7
	II	72	12.2	1386	5.8	41.1	640	1.1
	III	36	18.8	1441	6.0	43.7	850	1.3
3 children	I	34	6.7	1189	5.0	31.9	440	0.7
	II	73	12.1	1384	5.8	40.3	650	1.0
	III	38	19.9	1642	6.9	49.7	930	1.4
4 or more children	I	29	6.7	1262	5.3	34.2	450	0.8
	II	58	11.6	1443	6.0	40.9	630	1.1
	III	28	20.1	1735	7.3	52.3	970	1.4

[1]Group I: below 25th percentile milk intake.
Group II: between 25th and 75th percentile milk intake.
Group III: above 75th percentile milk intake.

Table A32: *Mean daily intake of energy and some nutrients of children aged 3½ and under 4½ years from families of different sizes in 3 groups[1] according to the intake of milk (oz) from all sources*

| Family size | Group | No. of children | Mean daily intake | | | | | |
			Milk oz	Energy kcal	Energy MJ	Total protein g	Calcium mg	Riboflavin mg
1–2 children	I	23	6.0	1244	5.2	33.4	430	0.8
	II	56	12.1	1345	5.6	38.8	620	1.0
	III	31	19.0	1692	7.1	50.5	920	1.4
3 children	I	30	6.9	1376	5.8	37.1	480	0.8
	II	67	11.7	1380	5.8	39.7	620	1.0
	III	22	17.6	1706	7.1	48.2	870	1.4
4 or more children	I	27	7.2	1293	5.4	34.2	460	0.8
	II	36	11.7	1526	6.4	42.4	650	1.1
	III	27	20.2	1884	7.9	55.2	990	1.6

[1]Group I: below 25th percentile milk intake.
Group II: between 25th and 75th percentile milk intake.
Group III: above 75th percentile milk intake.

Table A33: *Mean heights and weights (adjusted for age) of BOYS in four different age groups in the four quartiles[1] of total milk intake from all sources*

| Age group (years) | Quartiles[1] | Height | | | Weight | | |
		No. of children	Milk intake oz	Height cm	No. of children	Milk intake oz	Weight kg
½ and under 1½	All	103	16.3	75.7	104	16.3	10.9
	1	26	9.4	74.5	26	9.4	10.4
	2	26	13.9	75.9	26	13.9	10.8
	3	26	17.7	77.2	26	17.6	10.9
	4	25	24.6	75.4	26	24.4	11.3
1½ and under 2½	All	186	14.0	85.9	200	14.2	12.9
	1	47	7.7	85.4	50	7.6	12.4
	2	46	11.7	85.0	50	11.8	12.7
	3	47	14.9	86.4	50	15.0	12.9
	4	46	21.7	86.5	50	22.3	13.4
2½ and under 3½	All	188	12.9	94.3	195	12.8	14.7
	1	47	6.7	93.2	49	6.5	14.2
	2	47	11.0	94.5	49	11.0	14.7
	3	47	14.3	94.4	49	14.4	14.7
	4	47	19.6	94.9	48	19.6	15.4
3½ and under 4½	All	164	12.6	101.7	167	12.6	16.5
	1	41	6.8	102.4	42	6.8	16.7
	2	42	10.5	100.9	43	10.4	16.2
	3	40	13.5	100.7	41	13.5	16.1
	4	41	19.8	102.6	41	19.6	17.1

[1]Quartile 1: below 25th percentile milk intake.
Quartile 2: 25th–50th percentile milk intake.
Quartile 3: 50th–75th percentile milk intake.
Quartile 4: above 75th percentile milk intake.

Table A34: *Mean heights and weights (adjusted for age) of GIRLS in four different age groups in the four quartiles[1] of total milk intake from all sources*

Age group (years)	Quartiles[1]	Height			Weight		
		No. of children	Milk intake oz	Height cm	No. of children	Milk intake oz	Weight kg
$\frac{1}{2}$ and under $1\frac{1}{2}$	All	96	17.0	73.5	99	16.8	9.9
	1	24	8.1	74.1	25	8.0	9.9
	2	24	13.7	72.5	25	13.6	9.5
	3	24	17.5	74.0	24	17.5	10.2
	4	24	28.6	73.4	25	28.4	10.1
$1\frac{1}{2}$ and under $2\frac{1}{2}$	All	181	12.5	84.9	194	12.7	12.2
	1	45	7.1	83.9	48	7.1	11.9
	2	46	10.3	85.6	49	10.4	12.4
	3	45	13.3	85.8	48	13.5	12.5
	4	45	19.1	84.3	49	19.7	12.1
$2\frac{1}{2}$ and under $3\frac{1}{2}$	All	194	11.4	92.8	200	11.5	13.9
	1	48	5.8	91.9	50	5.8	13.4
	2	49	9.5	92.2	50	9.5	13.8
	3	48	12.3	94.2	50	12.4	14.3
	4	49	18.1	93.0	50	18.3	14.0
$3\frac{1}{2}$ and under $4\frac{1}{2}$	All	142	11.2	100.4	147	11.2	16.0
	1	35	5.9	100.2	36	5.9	15.9
	2	36	9.8	101.0	37	9.7	15.7
	3	35	12.1	99.4	37	12.0	16.2
	4	36	17.1	100.9	37	17.2	16.3

[1]Quartile 1: below 25th percentile milk intake.
Quartile 2: 25th–50th percentile milk intake.
Quartile 3: 50th–75th percentile milk intake.
Quartile 4: above 75th percentile milk intake.

61

Table A35: *Comparison of the mean daily intake of energy, "added sugars" and some nutrients of the 10 per cent of children with the lowest energy intake with those of all the children in the four age groups*

Age group (years)	No. of children	Mean daily intake					Percentage of energy from		
		Energy kcal	MJ	Protein g	Carbo-hydrate g	Total "added sugars"[1] g	Total protein	Total carbo-hydrate	Total "added sugars"[1]
½ and under 1½	Lowest 10%	660	2.8	23.5	90	33.8	14.3	34.4	20.4
	All	1050	4.4	33.9	141	48.0	12.9	50.3	18.3
1½ and under 2½	Lowest 10%	773	3.2	25.2	100	35.1	13.1	38.1	18.2
	All	1262	5.3	38.0	164	56.8	12.0	48.7	18.0
2½ and under 3½	Lowest 10%	889	3.7	27.1	117	42.7	12.2	37.7	19.2
	All	1401	5.9	40.7	186	64.7	11.6	49.7	18.5
3½ and under 4½	Lowest 10%	1006	4.2	28.8	138	53.0	11.5	37.0	20.7
	All	1468	6.1	41.6	197	69.4	11.3	50.4	18.9

[1] For definition see paragraph 3.2.3.

Table A36: *Comparison of mean daily energy and protein intake and height of all children and of the 10 per cent shortest children in the different age/sex groups*

Age group (years)	No. of children	Height adjusted for age cm	Energy kcal	Energy MJ	Protein g
BOYS					
½ and under 1½	All (103)	75.7	1053	4.4	33.7
	Below 10th percentile	66.7	1056	4.4	30.8
1½ and under 2½	All (186)	85.9	1273	5.3	38.5
	Below 10th percentile	78.3	1345	5.6	41.2
2½ and under 3½	All (188)	94.3	1466	6.1	42.3
	Below 10th percentile	84.2	1422	6.0	40.6
3½ and under 4½	All (164)	101.7	1534	6.4	44.0
	Below 10th percentile	93.7	1439	6.0	41.2
GIRLS					
½ and under 1½	All (96)	73.5	1049	4.4	34.5
	Below 10th percentile	66.3	1171	4.9	39.2
1½ and under 2½	All (181)	84.9	1237	5.2	37.0
	Below 10th percentile	77.3	1285	5.4	39.4
2½ and under 3½	All (194)	92.8	1326	5.6	38.7
	Below 10th percentile	82.6	1277	5.3	38.0
3½ and under 4½	All (142)	100.4	1404	5.9	39.7
	Below 10th percentile	92.0	1573	6.6	42.4

Table A37: *Comparison of mean daily energy and protein intake and weight of all children and of the 10 per cent lightest children in the different age/sex groups*

Age group (years)	No. of children	Weight¹ kg	Energy kcal	Energy MJ	Protein g
BOYS					
½ and under 1½	All (104)	10.9	1063	4.4	34.0
	Below 10th percentile	8.3	1066	4.5	33.4
1½ and under 2½	All (200)	12.9	1277	5.4	38.6
	Below 10th percentile	10.5	1255	5.3	35.8
2½ and under 3½	All (195)	14.7	1472	6.2	42.3
	Below 10th percentile	11.8	1231	5.2	35.7
3½ and under 4½	All (167)	16.5	1529	6.4	43.7
	Below 10th percentile	13.6	1433	6.0	42.5
GIRLS					
½ and under 1½	All (99)	10.1	1049	4.4	34.4
	Below 10th percentile	7.7	989	4.1	32.9
1½ and under 2½	All (194)	12.2	1235	5.2	37.1
	Below 10th percentile	9.9	1242	5.2	35.9
2½ and under 3½	All (200)	13.9	1335	5.6	39.0
	Below 10th percentile	11.0	1232	5.2	35.0
3½ and under 4½	All (147)	16.0	1409	5.9	39.8
	Below 10th percentile	13.1	1534	6.4	44.3

¹ Weight adjusted for age.

Table A.38: *Comparison of mean daily intake of energy, protein, carbohydrate, "added sugars"[1] and Quetelet's index[2] of all children, those with Quetelet's index below the 10th percentile and those with Quetelet's index above the 90th percentile in the different age/sex groups*

Age group (years)	No. of children	Quetelet's Index[2]	Energy kcal	MJ	Protein g	Total carbohydrate g	"Added sugars"[1] g
BOYS							
½ and under 1½	All (102)	1.9	1056	4.4	33.8	145	52.3
	Below 10 percentile	1.6	1020	4.3	34.7	138	47.4
	Above 90 percentile	2.4	990	4.1	32.2	136	50.0
1½ and under 2½	All (186)	1.8	1273	5.3	38.5	165	56.7
	Below 10th percentile	1.5	1162	4.9	33.6	151	52.6
	Above 90th percentile	2.1	1417	5.9	42.9	184	61.1
2½ and under 3½	All (186)	1.7	1465	6.1	42.2	195	68.4
	Below 10th percentile	1.4	1354	5.7	38.6	180	66.2
	Above 90th percentile	2.2	1574	6.6	43.7	213	76.1
3½ and under 4½	All (163)	1.6	1528	6.4	43.7	205	70.9
	Below 10th percentile	1.4	1442	6.0	41.0	193	71.7
	Above 90th percentile	1.9	1746	7.3	49.5	229	78.7
GIRLS							
½ and under 1½	All (96)	1.8	1048	4.4	34.5	135	40.7
	Below 10th percentile	1.5	951	4.0	31.9	121	40.3
	Above 90th percentile	2.3	1275	5.3	41.5	156	45.5
1½ and under 2½	All(179)	1.7	1235	5.2	37.0	161	56.5
	Below 10th percentile	1.4	1286	5.4	36.8	164	56.9
	Above 90th percentile	2.1	1237	5.2	39.0	156	50.2
2½ and under 3½	All (191)	1.6	1327	5.6	38.7	175	61.2
	Below 10th percentile	1.4	1205	5.0	34.2	163	56.3
	Above 90th percentile	2.0	1289	5.4	39.6	166	53.2
3½ and under 4½	All (142)	1.6	1404	5.9	39.7	188	66.4
	Below 10th percentile	1.3	1276	5.3	35.9	176	63.6
	Above 90th percentile	2.0	1415	5.9	39.0	192	69.2

[1]For definition see paragraph 3.2.3.

[2]Quetelet's index = $\dfrac{\text{Weight (kg)}}{\text{Height (cm)}^2} \times 1000$.

Table A39: *Standard deviations of mean height in this study compared with values from 8 other countries*

Age (years)	This survey[1]	Switzerland	France	Germany	Norway	Czechoslovakia	England	USA	China
BOYS									
1	4.6	—	—	—	—	—	—	—	—
2	4.1	4.1	2.8	3.5	3.9	—	3.5	3.5	—
3	5.4	4.1	5.7	4.0	4.1	4.4	4.2	3.4	3.5
4	5.0	4.3	4.5	4.0	4.8	4.5	4.0	3.9	3.9
GIRLS									
1	3.7	—	—	—	—	—	—	—	—
2	3.8	3.9	3.7	3.5	4.1	—	2.7	2.9	—
3	4.9	4.3	5.1	3.5	4.7	4.4	3.5	3.4	3.9
4	4.7	4.5	3.7	4.0	4.3	4.6	3.7	4.0	4.6

SOURCE: Heimendinger (1964).

[1]See footnote to Table A40.

Table A40: *Standard deviations of mean weight in this study compared with values from 8 other countries*

Age (years)	This survey[1]	Switzerland	France	Germany	Norway	Czechoslovakia	England	USA	China
BOYS									
1	1.4	—	—	—	—	—	—	—	—
2	1.5	2.0	1.2	1.3	1.4	—	1.2	1.3	—
3	1.8	2.1	1.4	1.5	1.4	1.7	1.5	1.5	1.7
4	2.0	2.0	1.6	1.7	1.9	1.8	1.9	1.7	1.4
GIRLS									
1	1.4	—	—	—	—	—	—	—	—
2	1.5	1.4	1.2	1.3	1.4	—	1.2	1.3	—
3	1.8	2.0	1.4	1.9	1.8	1.7	1.4	1.6	1.5
4	1.9	2.3	1.6	1.7	1.8	2.0	1.5	2.0	1.5

SOURCE: Heimendinger (1964).

[1]Heights and weights were adjusted to the mid-points of the age ranges in the 4 groups $\frac{1}{2}$ and under $1\frac{1}{2}$ years, $1\frac{1}{2}$ and under $2\frac{1}{2}$ years, $2\frac{1}{2}$ and under $3\frac{1}{2}$ years and $3\frac{1}{2}$ and under $4\frac{1}{2}$ years.

Table A41: *Mean daily intake of energy and nutrients of children who had a medical examination and those who did not in the 1967–68 survey, and those who had a medical examination in the 1963 survey (number of children in parentheses)*

Nutrient		Children who had a full medical examination		Children who had no examination
		1963 (337)	1967–68 (95)	1967–68 (1226)
Energy	kcal	1269	1304	1324
	MJ	5.4	5.5	5.5
Protein	g	37.7	40.2	39.0
Fat	g	56	55	56
Total carbohydrate	g	163	172	175
"Added sugars"[1]	g	53.0	61.8	60.9
Calcium	mg	720	670	690
Iron	mg	7.3	6.7	6.9
Vitamin A	iu	2290	2260	2440
	µg	690	680	730
Thiamin	mg	0.7	0.6	0.7
Riboflavin	mg	1.1	1.1	1.1
Nicotinic acid	mg	5.8	7.1	7.1
Vitamin C	mg	28	41	40
Vitamin D	iu	126	79	112
	µg	3.2	2.0	2.8
Pyridoxine	mg	0.6	0.7	0.6
Percentage calories from protein		12.0	12.5	11.9

[1] For definition see paragraph 3.2.3.

Table A42: *List of food groups*

01: Manufactured baby foods, rusks.
02: Food supplements (welfare).
03: Food supplements (other than welfare).
04: Breakfast cereals.
05: Other cereals.
06: Bread.
07: Biscuits, cakes and pastries, flour confectionery, puddings, tarts and fruit dishes made with pastry, etc.
08: Sugar and preserves.
09: Confectionery.
10: Potatoes.
11: Green vegetables and tomatoes.
12: Pulses, root and miscellaneous vegetables.
13: Raw fruits, citrus.
14: Raw fruits, other than citrus.
15: Fruits—tinned, bottled and dried, and fruit juices.
16: Liver.
17: Meat (other than liver) and meat dishes.
18: Fish and fish dishes.
19: Eggs and egg dishes.
20: Cheese and cheese dishes.
21: Milk—liquid forms.
22: Milk—dried baby milks.
23: Fats and oils.
24: Not used.
25: Alcohol.
26: All other items.

Diagram A1 : *Percentage contribution of some food groups to the dietary intake of energy*

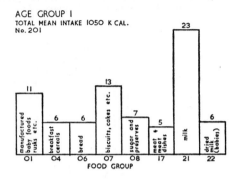

AGE GROUP I
TOTAL MEAN INTAKE 1050 K CAL.
No. 201

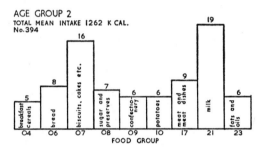

AGE GROUP 2
TOTAL MEAN INTAKE 1262 K CAL.
No. 394

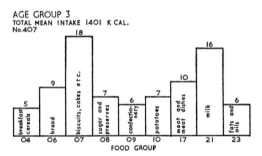

AGE GROUP 3
TOTAL MEAN INTAKE 1401 K CAL.
No. 407

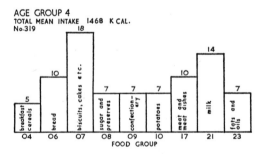

AGE GROUP 4
TOTAL MEAN INTAKE 1468 K CAL.
No. 319

68

Diagram A2: *Percentage contribution of some food groups to the dietary intake of total protein*

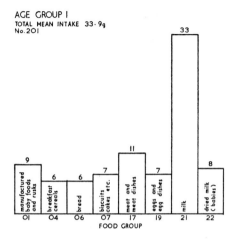

AGE GROUP 1
TOTAL MEAN INTAKE 33·9g
No.201

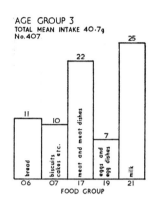

AGE GROUP 3
TOTAL MEAN INTAKE 40·7g
No.407

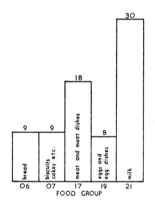

AGE GROUP 2
TOTAL MEAN INTAKE 38·0g
No.394

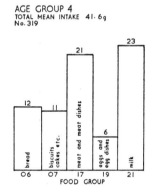

AGE GROUP 4
TOTAL MEAN INTAKE 41·6g
No.319

69

Diagram A3: *Percentage contribution of some food groups to the dietary intake of fat*

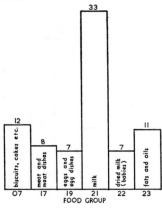

AGE GROUP 1
TOTAL MEAN INTAKE 42·6g
No. 201

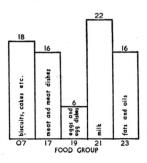

AGE GROUP 3
TOTAL MEAN INTAKE 59·7g
No. 407

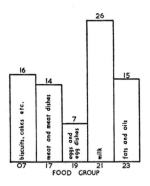

AGE GROUP 2
TOTAL MEAN INTAKE 54·4g
No. 394

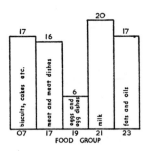

AGE GROUP 4
TOTAL MEAN INTAKE 61·9g
No. 319

Diagram A4: *Percentage contribution of some food groups to the dietary intake of total carbohydrate*

AGE GROUP 1
TOTAL MEAN INTAKE 140·8g
No.201

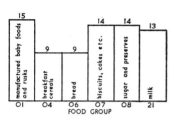

AGE GROUP 3
TOTAL MEAN INTAKE 185·7g
No.407

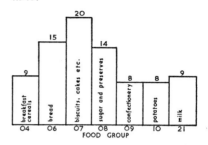

AGE GROUP 2
TOTAL MEAN INTAKE 164·0g
No.394

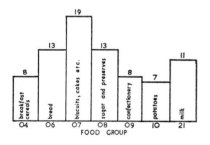

AGE GROUP 4
TOTAL MEAN INTAKE 197·2g
No.319

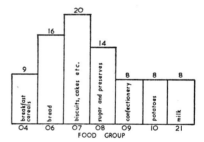

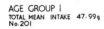

Diagram A5: *Percentage contribution of some food groups to the dietary intake of "added sugars"*

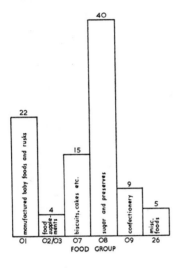

AGE GROUP I
TOTAL MEAN INTAKE 47·99g
No. 201

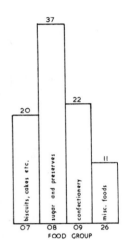

AGE GROUP 3
TOTAL MEAN INTAKE 64·72g
No. 407

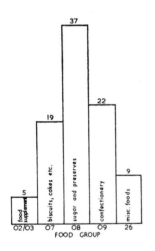

AGE GROUP 2
TOTAL MEAN INTAKE 56·78g
No. 394

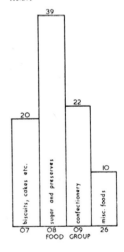

AGE GROUP 4
TOTAL MEAN INTAKE 69·35g
No. 319

Diagram A6: *Percentage contribution of some food groups to the dietary intake of calcium*

AGE GROUP 1
TOTAL MEAN INTAKE 771·2 mg
No. 201

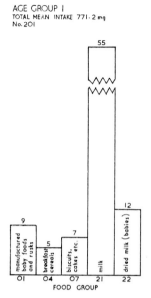

FOOD GROUP

AGE GROUP 3
TOTAL MEAN INTAKE 658·2 mg
No. 407

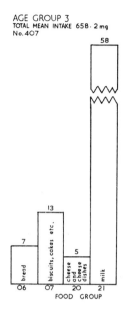

FOOD GROUP

AGE GROUP 2
TOTAL MEAN INTAKE 691·4 mg
No. 394

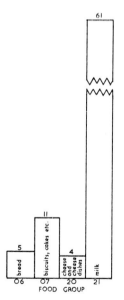

FOOD GROUP

AGE GROUP 4
TOTAL MEAN INTAKE 661·3 mg
No. 319

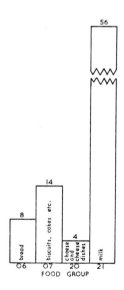

FOOD GROUP

73

Diagram A7: *Percentage contribution of some food groups to the dietary intake of iron*

AGE GROUP 1.
TOTAL MEAN INTAKE 7·64mg
No. 201.

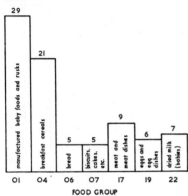

AGE GROUP 3.
TOTAL MEAN INTAKE 6·78mg
No. 407

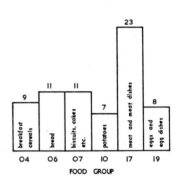

AGE GROUP 2.
TOTAL MEAN INTAKE 6·56 mg
No. 394.

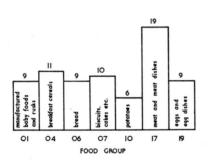

AGE GROUP 4.
TOTAL MEAN INTAKE 7·08 mg
No. 319.

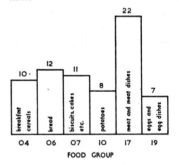

Diagram A8: *Percentage contribution of some food groups to the dietary intake of thiamin*

AGE GROUP 1.
TOTAL MEAN INTAKE 0·641mg
No.201.

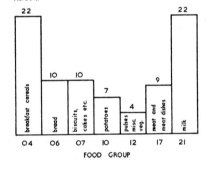

AGE GROUP 3.
TOTAL MEAN INTAKE 0·672mg
No.407.

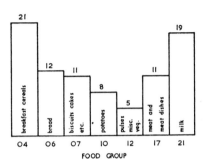

AGE GROUP 2.
TOTAL MEAN INTAKE 0·622mg
No.394.

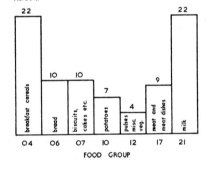

AGE GROUP 4.
TOTAL MEAN INTAKE 0·701mg
No.319.

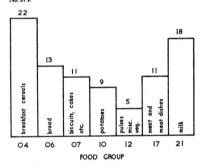

75

Diagram A9: *Percentage contribution of some food groups to the dietary intake of riboflavin*

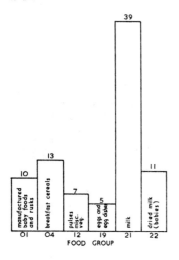

AGE GROUP 1
TOTAL MEAN INTAKE 1·250 mg.
No. 201

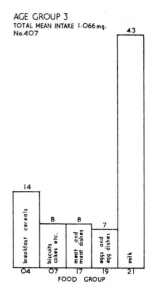

AGE GROUP 3
TOTAL MEAN INTAKE 1·066 mg.
No. 407

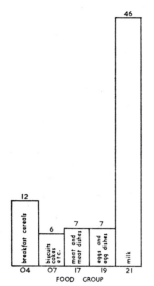

AGE GROUP 2
TOTAL MEAN INTAKE 1·069 mg
No. 394

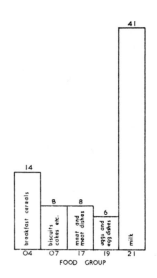

AGE GROUP 4
TOTAL MEAN INTAKE 1·083 mg
No. 319

Diagram A10: *Percentage contribution of some food groups to the dietary intake of vitamin A*

AGE GROUP 1
TOTAL MEAN INTAKE 2762 i.u.
No.201

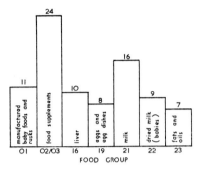

AGE GROUP 3
TOTAL MEAN INTAKE 2224 i.u.
No.407

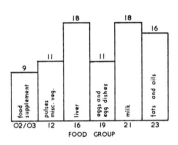

AGE GROUP 2
TOTAL MEAN INTAKE 2505 i.u.
No.394

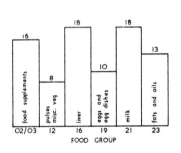

AGE GROUP 4
TOTAL MEAN INTAKE 2391 i.u.
No.319

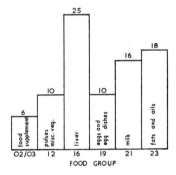

77

Diagram A11 : *Percentage contribution of some food groups to the dietary intake of vitamin C*

AGE GROUP 1.
TOTAL MEAN INTAKE 46·7 mg
No. 201.

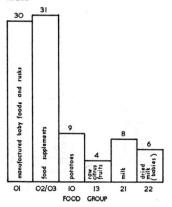

AGE GROUP 3.
TOTAL MEAN INTAKE 36·8 mg
No. 407.

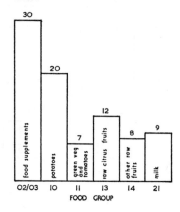

AGE GROUP 2.
TOTAL MEAN INTAKE 40·3 mg
No. 394.

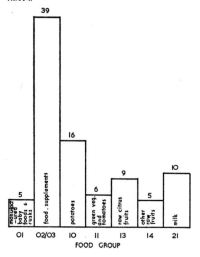

AGE GROUP 4.
TOTAL MEAN INTAKE 37·7 mg
No. 319.

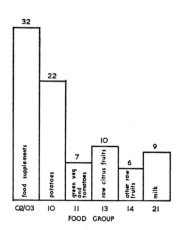

Diagram A12: *Percentage contribution of some food groups to the dietary intake of vitamin D*

AGE GROUP 1.
TOTAL MEAN INTAKE 215·3 i.u.
No. 201.

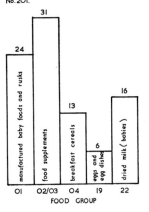

AGE GROUP 3.
TOTAL MEAN INTAKE 80·6 i.u.
No. 407.

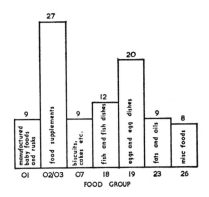

AGE GROUP 2.
TOTAL MEAN INTAKE 114·6 i.u.
No. 394.

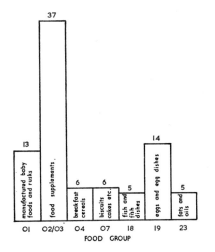

AGE GROUP 4.
TOTAL MEAN INTAKE 72·7 i.u.
No. 319

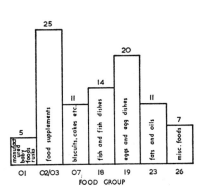

79

Diagram A13: *Percentage frequency distribution of mean daily intakes of milk*[1] *(Percentage of children per 2.5 oz intake group given at the head of each column)*

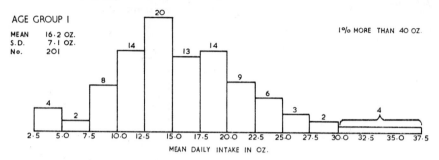

AGE GROUP 1

MEAN   16·2 OZ.
S.D.   7·1 OZ.
No.   201

1% MORE THAN 40 OZ.

MEAN DAILY INTAKE IN OZ.

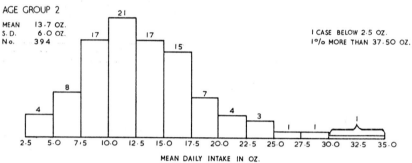

AGE GROUP 2

MEAN   13·7 OZ.
S.D.   6·0 OZ.
No.   394

1 CASE BELOW 2·5 OZ.
1% MORE THAN 37·50 OZ.

MEAN DAILY INTAKE IN OZ.

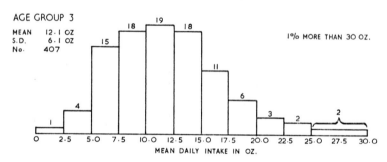

AGE GROUP 3

MEAN   12·1 OZ
S.D.   6·1 OZ
No.   407

1% MORE THAN 30 OZ.

MEAN DAILY INTAKE IN OZ.

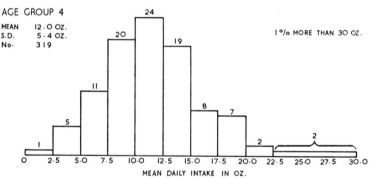

AGE GROUP 4

MEAN   12·0 OZ.
S.D.   5·4 OZ.
No·   319

1% MORE THAN 30 OZ.

MEAN DAILY INTAKE IN OZ.

[1] Milk, for the purpose of these diagrams, includes all types of milk—fresh, full and half-cream dried milk and evaporated milk—from all sources (drunk as milk, milk used in puddings, ice-cream etc.). The weights of both evaporated and dried milk have been converted to a liquid equivalent. A small amount of dried skimmed milk has not been included. This amount averages 0.2–0.4 oz per day.

Diagram A14: *Percentage frequency distribution of mean daily intakes of meat*[1]

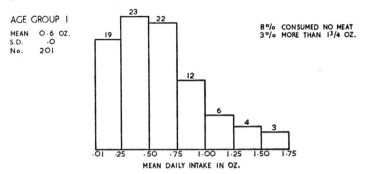

AGE GROUP I

MEAN 0·6 OZ.
S.D.   ·O
No.   201

8% CONSUMED NO MEAT
3% MORE THAN 1³/4 OZ.

MEAN DAILY INTAKE IN OZ.

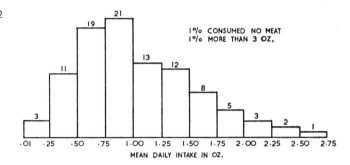

AGE GROUP 2

MEAN 1·1 OZ
S.D.   ·O
No.   394

1% CONSUMED NO MEAT
1% MORE THAN 3 OZ.

MEAN DAILY INTAKE IN OZ.

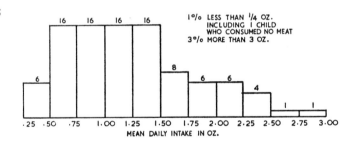

AGE GROUP 3

MEAN 1·3 OZ
S.D.   ·O
No.   407

1% LESS THAN ¹/4 OZ.
INCLUDING 1 CHILD
WHO CONSUMED NO MEAT
3% MORE THAN 3 OZ.

MEAN DAILY INTAKE IN OZ.

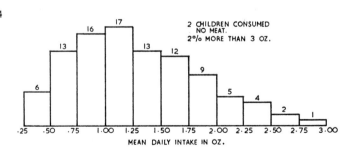

AGE GROUP 4

MEAN 1·3 OZ.
S.D.   ·O
No.   319

2 CHILDREN CONSUMED
NO MEAT.
2% MORE THAN 3 OZ.

MEAN DAILY INTAKE IN OZ.

[1] Meat, for the purpose of these diagrams, includes meat from all sources (roast, grilled etc. and meat in meat pies etc.).

Diagram A15: *Mean daily energy intakes of children in four different age groups in the four quarters of the year*

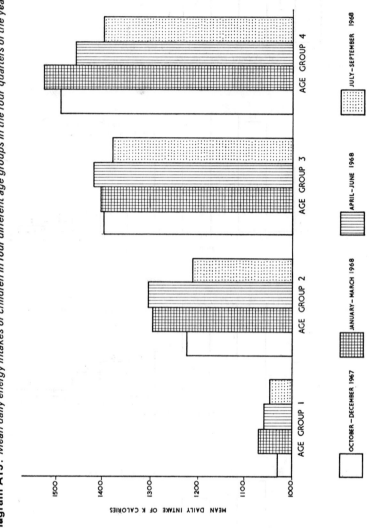

Diagram A16 : *Percentage frequency distribution of mean daily intakes of energy[1] (Percentage of children per 200 kcal intake group given at head of each column)*

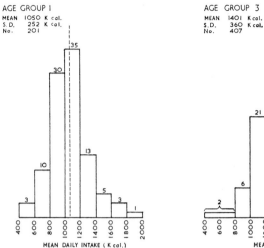

AGE GROUP 1

MEAN 1050 K cal.
S.D. 252 K cal.
No. 201

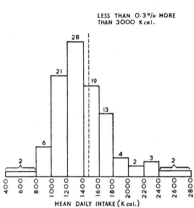

AGE GROUP 3

MEAN 1401 Kcal.
S.D. 360 Kcal.
No. 407

LESS THAN 0.3% MORE
THAN 3000 Kcal.

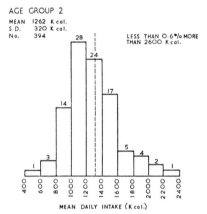

AGE GROUP 2

MEAN 1262 K cal.
S.D. 320 K cal.
No. 394

LESS THAN 0.6% MORE
THAN 2600 Kcal.

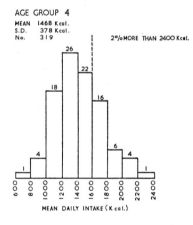

AGE GROUP 4

MEAN 1468 Kcal.
S.D. 378 Kcal.
No. 319

2% MORE THAN 2400 Kcal.

[1] The recommended daily intake estimated as being appropriate to children at the mid-point of the age group is shown by the vertical broken line.

83

Diagram A17: *Percentage frequency distribution of mean daily intakes of total protein[1]*
(Percentage of children per 5 g intake group given at the head of each
column)

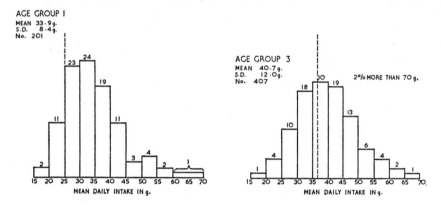

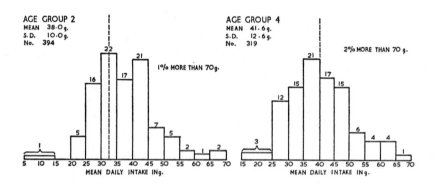

[1] The recommended daily intake estimated as being appropriate to children at the mid-point of the age group is shown by the vertical dotted line.

Diagram A18: *Percentage frequency distribution of mean daily intakes of calcium[1]*
(Percentage of children per 200 mg intake group given at the head of each
column)

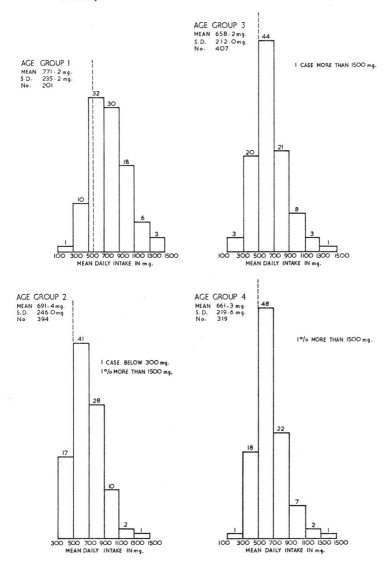

AGE GROUP 3
MEAN 658.2 mg.
S.D. 212.0 mg.
No.   407

I CASE MORE THAN 1500 mg.

AGE GROUP I
MEAN 771.2 mg.
S.D. 235.2 mg.
No.   201

32

30

18

10

6

3

1

100 300 500 700 900 1100 1300 1500
MEAN DAILY INTAKE IN mg.

44

20

21

8

3

3

1

100 300 500 700 900 1100 1300 1500
MEAN DAILY INTAKE IN mg.

AGE GROUP 2
MEAN 691.4 mg.
S.D. 246.0 mg
No.   394

41

I CASE BELOW 300 mg.
1% MORE THAN 1500 mg.

28

17

10

2

1

300 500 700 900 1100 1300 1500
MEAN DAILY INTAKE IN mg.

AGE GROUP 4
MEAN 661.3 mg.
S.D. 219.6 mg.
No.   319

48

1% MORE THAN 1500 mg.

22

18

7

2

1

1

100 300 500 700 900 1100 1300 1500
MEAN DAILY INTAKE IN mg.

[1]The recommended daily intake estimated as being appropriate to children at the mid-point of the age group
is shown by the vertical dotted line.

85

Diagram A19: *Percentage frequency distribution of mean daily intakes of iron[1] (Percentage of children per mg intake group given at the head of each column)*

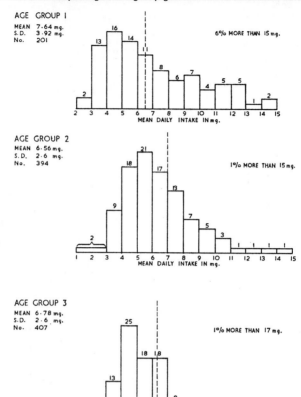

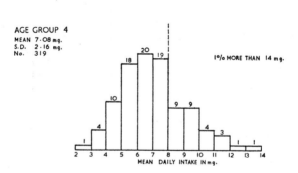

[1]The recommended daily intake estimated as being appropriate to children at the mid-point of the age group is shown by the vertical dotted line.

Diagram A20: *Percentage frequency distribution of mean daily intakes of riboflavin* [1]
(Percentage of children per 0.2 mg intake group given at the head of each column)

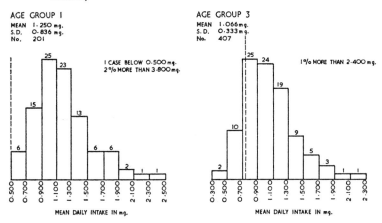

AGE GROUP I

MEAN   1.250 mg.
S.D.   0.836 mg.
No.   201

I CASE BELOW 0.500 mg.
2% MORE THAN 3.800 mg.

MEAN DAILY INTAKE IN mg.

AGE GROUP 3

MEAN   1.066 mg.
S.D.   0.333 mg.
No.   407

1% MORE THAN 2.400 mg.

MEAN DAILY INTAKE IN mg.

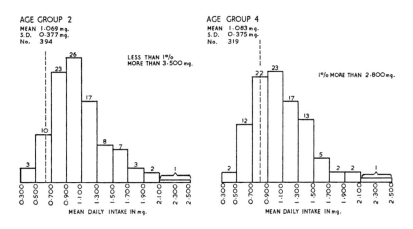

AGE GROUP 2

MEAN   1.069 mg.
S.D.   0.377 mg.
No.   394

LESS THAN 1%
MORE THAN 3.500 mg.

MEAN DAILY INTAKE IN mg.

AGE GROUP 4

MEAN   1.083 mg.
S.D.   0.375 mg.
No.   319

1% MORE THAN 2.800 mg.

MEAN DAILY INTAKE IN mg.

[1] The recommended daily intake estimated as being appropriate to children at the mid-point of the age group is shown by the vertical dotted line.

87

Diagram A21: *Percentage frequency distribution of mean daily intakes of vitamin C[1]*
(Percentage of children per 10 mg intake group given at the head of each
column)

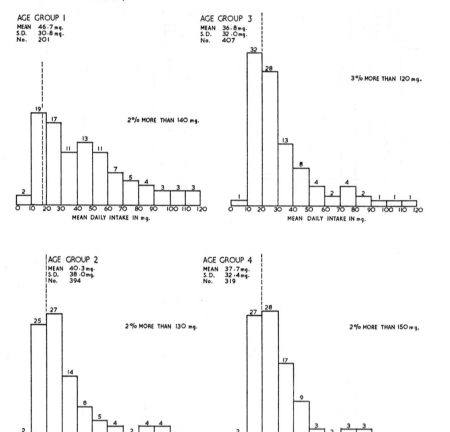

AGE GROUP 1
MEAN 46·7 mg.
S.D. 30·8 mg.
No. 201

2% MORE THAN 140 mg.

MEAN DAILY INTAKE IN mg.

AGE GROUP 3
MEAN 36·8 mg.
S.D. 32·0 mg.
No. 407

3% MORE THAN 120 mg.

MEAN DAILY INTAKE IN mg.

AGE GROUP 2
MEAN 40·3 mg.
S.D. 38·0 mg.
No. 394

2% MORE THAN 130 mg.

MEAN DAILY INTAKE IN mg.

AGE GROUP 4
MEAN 37·7 mg.
S.D. 32·4 mg.
No. 319

2% MORE THAN 150 mg.

MEAN DAILY INTAKE IN mg.

[1]The recommended daily intake estimated as being appropriate to children at the mid-point of the age group
is shown by the vertical dotted line.

88

Diagram A22: *Percentage frequency distribution of mean daily intakes of vitamin D (Percentage of children per 25 iu intake group given at the head of each column)*

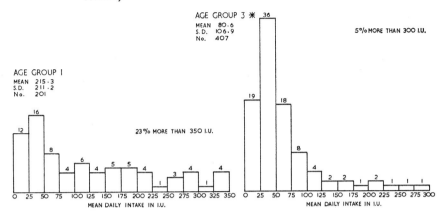

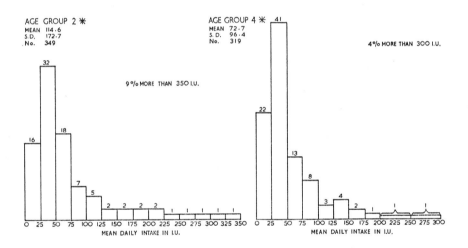

*The standard deviation was distended by a few children with very high intakes of vitamin D and was greater than the mean in these groups.

89

Diagram A23: *Percentage frequency distribution of mean daily intakes of total "added sugars"[1] (Percentage of children per 10 g intake group given at the head of each column)*

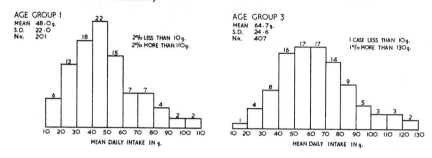

AGE GROUP 1
MEAN 48·0 g.
S.D. 22·0
No. 201

2% LESS THAN 10g.
2% MORE THAN 110g.

MEAN DAILY INTAKE IN g.

AGE GROUP 3
MEAN 64·7 g.
S.D. 24·6
No. 407

1 CASE LESS THAN 10g.
1% MORE THAN 130g.

MEAN DAILY INTAKE IN g.

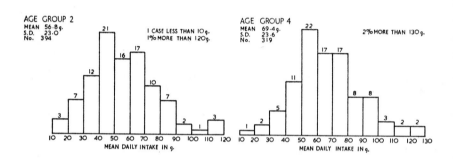

AGE GROUP 2
MEAN 56·8 g.
S.D. 23·0
No. 394

1 CASE LESS THAN 10g.
1% MORE THAN 120g.

MEAN DAILY INTAKE IN g.

AGE GROUP 4
MEAN 69·4 g.
S.D. 23·6
No. 319

2% MORE THAN 130g.

MEAN DAILY INTAKE IN g.

[1] For definition see para. 3.2.3

90

Diagram A24: *Scatter diagrams showing the relationship between the mean daily energy intake and the recommended daily intake[1] of energy in (a) boys of different ages, and (b) girls of different ages*

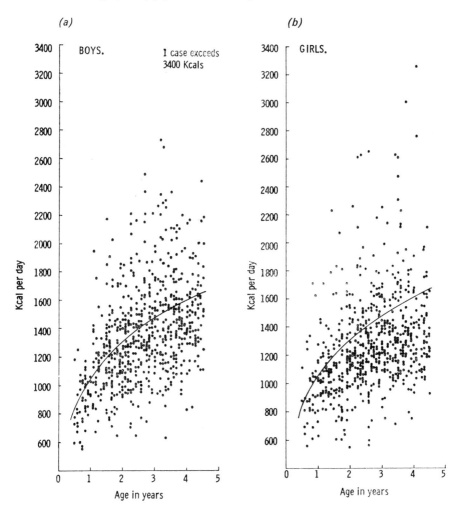

[1]The line represents the recommended daily intake of energy for boys and girls of different ages.

Diagram A25: *Percentage frequency distribution of height (cm) adjusted for age in*

(a) Boys and girls aged ½ and under 1½ years

(c) Boys and girls aged 2½ and under 3½ years

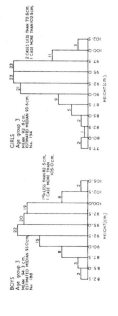

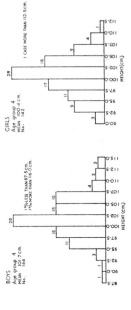

(b) Boys and girls aged 1½ and under 2½ years

(d) Boys and girls aged 3½ and under 4½ years

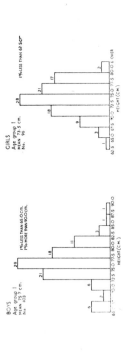

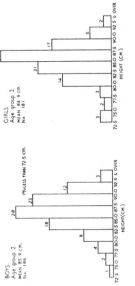

Diagram A26: *Percentage frequency distribution of weight (kg) adjusted for age in*

(a) Boys and girls aged ½ and under 1½ years

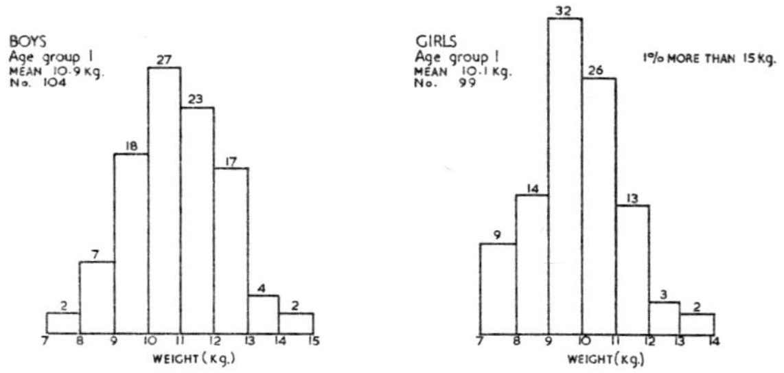

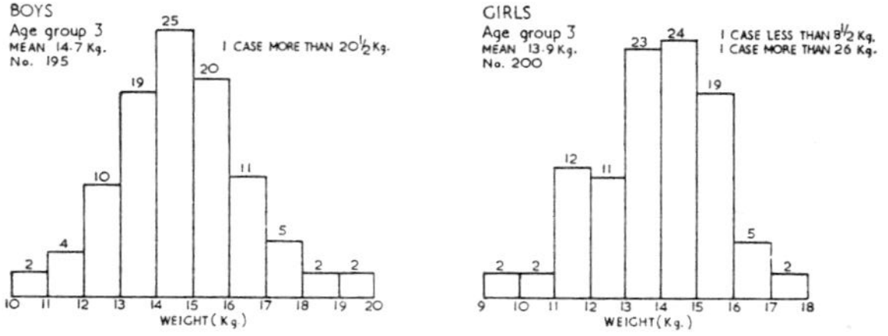

(b) Boys and girls aged 1½ and under 2½ years

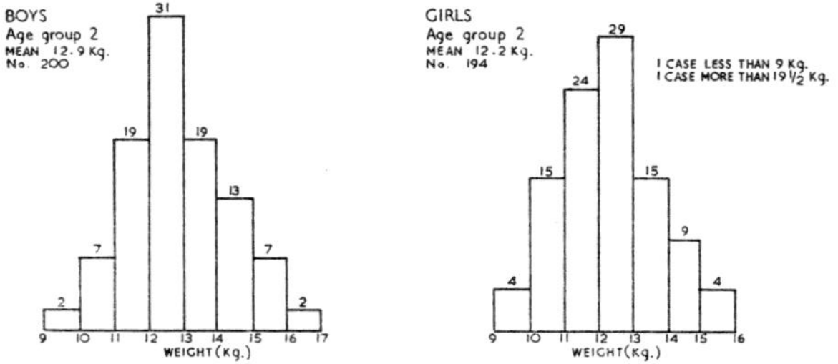

(c) Boys and girls aged 2½ and under 3½ years

(d) Boys and girls aged 3½ and under 4½ years

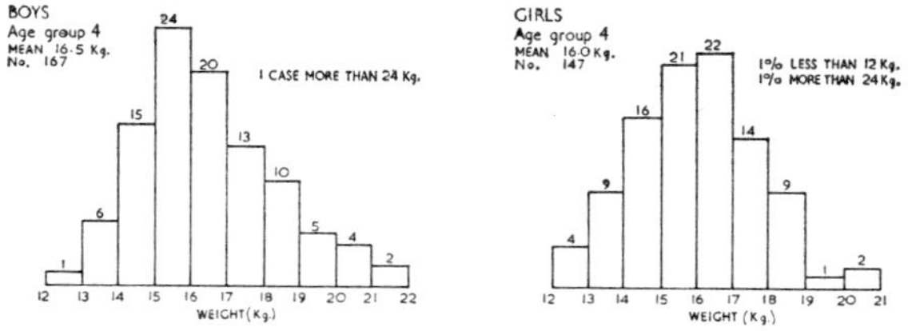

93

14. Appendix B
Forms used in the survey

For a detailed list, see p xvi

B1-Nutrition Survey (Young Children)

CONTACT SHEET

STAT NS/12
J.N. 46156

TRANSFER FROM ADDRESS LIST:

Local Authority Area_____

Name of child_____

Date of birth_____ Area Code

Name of mother or guardian_____

Address_____ Child Serial Number

_____

_____

Interviewer_____ Code No._____

RECORD OF CONTACT/PLACING CALLS

DATE	TIME	RESULT OF CALL

APPOINTMENTS, CHECKING AND COLLECTING CALLS

APPOINTMENT FOR:		CHECK OR COLLECTION ACTUALLY MADE		NOTES	DIARY CHECKED		BALANCE CHECKED
Date	Time	Date	Time		(i)	(ii)	

N.B. DIARY CHECKING: Col (i) is for checking unrecorded meals, eaten away from home, etc.

Col (ii) is for other checks to be completed as indicated in STAT NS/13 Appendix.

TRANSFER FROM CONTACT SHEET:

Area Code

Child Serial No.

Child's Date of Birth _____

Date of Interview _____ /196
          (Month)   (Year)

OUTCOME OF FINAL CONTACT CALL

Mother or guardian contacted 1

Child moved away 2

Child temporarily away 3

Child dead 4

Child not known at this address 5

No contact because mother not at home after 1 visit 6

                                   2 visits................7

                                   3 visits................8

Contact not made for other reasons...9

OUTCOME OF ATTEMPT TO INTERVIEW

Refused to be interviewed 1

Not interviewed because of language problem 2

Contacted but interview not completed because child
   at school/wrong age/breast-fed 3

Contacted but interview not completed (child in
   hospital/on holiday/moving) 4

Interviewed but could not keep record (will be away/
   in hospital) 5

Interviewed but refused to keep record 6

Interviewed and agreed to keep record 7

OFFICE USE ONLY	
	1–2
	3–4
	5
	6
	7
	8–10
	11
	12–14
	15

CONTACT QUESTIONNAIRE

INTRODUCTION

I am from the British Market Research Bureau, and am calling on behalf of the Ministry of Health/Scottish Home and Health Department/Welsh Board of Health, who would like to find out what kind of food and how much food young children eat. Any information you give will be used for statistical purposes and your name and address is known only to the British Market Research Bureau, the Government Social Survey and the Ministry of Health (or the Health Department for Scotland and Wales) who will use it only in connection with the present survey or in any enquiry of a medical, dental or nutritional nature following on this one. Your identity will not be revealed outside the organisations just mentioned, or in any publication of the results of this survey.

DO **NOT** MENTION BOOK OR WEIGHING.

1 (a) I'd like to talk to you about your son/daughter.................................(name of sample child)

IF THIS CHILD DOES NOT LIVE AT THIS ADDRESS CLOSE INTERVIEW.

(b) What is his/her date of birth?_____/_____/19____

IF THIS DATE DOES NOT FALL WITHIN THE TWO DATES YOU HAVE BEEN GIVEN FOR THE MONTH IN WHICH YOU ARE WORKING CLOSE INTERVIEW.

2   Does he/she attend a nursery or a day school of any kind?

Yes
No

IF "Yes" CLOSE INTERVIEW
IF "CHILD IS UNDER 2 YEARS OLD":

3(a) Is he/she fully weaned?

Yes
No

IF "No":

(b) Is he/she breast-fed or bottle fed?

Breast-fed
Bottle-fed
Both

IF "Breast-fed" OR "Both" CLOSE INTERVIEW.

IF CHILD IS ELIGIBLE GO TO MAIN QUESTIONNAIRE. DO NOT PRESS FOR ANSWERS TO ANY QUESTIONS AT THE RISK OF LOSING CO-OPERATION OVER KEEPING RECORD.

HOUSEHOLD COMPOSITION

4 Can you tell me who else there is in your household living there besides yourself? (I don't mean people who cater for themselves separately.) First your family and relatives. Include adopted, foster and step-children but no-one permanently living away from home.

FAMILY UNIT

Code No.	Relationship to respondent	Sex M	F	Age last birth- day	NORMAL occupational status Has paid job Full time 30 +	Part time	No paid job
1	RESPONDENT						
2	SELECTED CHILD						
3							
4							
5							
6							
7							
8							

Is there anyone else, **not** related to you, who is a member of the household living here, that is, who does not cater for themselves separately?

OTHER MEMBERS OF HOUSEHOLD

9							
10							
11							
12							
13							
14							
15							
16							

OFFICE USE ONLY

16

17

18

19

20

21

22–24

Questions 5 and 6 are to be asked about the husband of the mother of the selected child. If there is NO husband, they are to be asked about the mother (or guardian) of the child.

5(a) What is husband's/your occupation (if unemployed, sick or retired, indicate which and give former occupation)

....

(b) Is/was he/you self-employed? Yes.............No.............

(c) If "No" to (b), by what type of organisation is/was he/you employed (e.g. private firm, local government, civil service)?

....

(d) What grade or type of position does/did he/you hold (manager, foreman, apprentice, trainee, etc.)?

....

98

6(a) What is your husband's (your) **gross** weekly/monthly/yearly income—that is **before** deduction of income tax, national insurance, etc.?

Weekly £ _____

Monthly £ _____

Annual £ _____

STATE WHETHER: Actual	1
OR	
Estimated	2
Don't know/refused	3

This is his/your income before anything is deducted isn't it?

Yes	4
No	5

IF "Gross income given is more than £11 per week" GO TO Q.8.

IF "Gross income given is less than £11 per week"

(b) Is there any other member of your household who earns more than this?

Yes	1
No	2

IF "No" GO TO Q.8.

IF "Yes"

(c) Who is that (RECORD PERSON NUMBER FROM HOUSEHOLD COMPOSITION BOX)

IF "More than one person in this category"

(d) Which of these earns most? (RECORD PERSON NUMBER)

7 What is his/her **gross** weekly/monthly/yearly income— that is, **before** deduction of income tax, national insurance, etc.?

Weekly £ _____

Monthly £ _____

Annual £ _____

STATE WHETHER: Actual	1
OR	
Estimated	2
Don't know/refused	3

This is his/her income **before** anything is deducted isn't it?

Yes	4
No	5

8   How old were you when you finished your
full-time education?

	15 or under	1
	16–18	2
	19 or over	3

9(a) In what country were you born? _____

IF "Not Great Britain (i.e. England, Wales, Scotland)"

(b) How long have you been living in Great Britain?

_____

10(a) Is your child's feeding or choice of foods affected by any
medical condition?

Yes	1
No	2

IF "No" GO TO Q.11.
IF "Yes"

(b) What is the nature of this condition?

_____

_____

(c) And how is feeding affected?

_____

_____

(d) For how long has he/she had this condition?

_____

_____

11   Would you give me details about any particular foods
which your child does not eat for health or other reasons?

Food	Reason
_____	_____
_____	_____
_____	_____
_____	_____
_____	_____
_____	_____
_____	_____

100

Now give the mother a copy of the hand-out notice and ask her if she would be willing to keep a weighed dietary record for a week, assuring her that her name will not be published in connection with any of the information given.

Mother agrees	1
Does not agree	2

IF MOTHER DOES NOT AGREE, STATE REASON:

....

....

....

AND GO TO QUESTIONS 12, 13, 16 AND 17

IF MOTHER AGREES TO KEEP RECORD, HAND OVER RECORD BOOK, NOTEBOOK AND SCALES AND EXPLAIN FOLLOWING:

1. Child should have his/her usual meals.

2. **All** the food eaten should be recorded and examples of how this should be done are shown in the record book. Explain any other points from the record book if necessary.

3. The section about bed-times (and milk purchases) should be completed **every** day.

4. Give demonstration of cumulative weighing and let the mother do a trial weighing in your presence, filling in the back page of the record book.

5. Check the balance.

6. Ask the mother to start keeping a record book when the child next has something to eat (even if only a snack).

THEN ARRANGE AN APPOINTMENT FOR THE FIRST CHECKING CALL AND CLOSE THE INTERVIEW.

	OFFICE USE ONLY

12 May I weigh and measure your child?

Yes 1

No 2   29–31

IF "Yes" RECORD DETAILS BELOW

Height of child (without shoes)_____cms.   32–35
                 (to nearest whole number)

Weight of child   _____lbs.
                 (to nearest quarter lb.)   36–38

Fully clothed 1

Partially clothed 2   39–41

13 May I measure your height at the same time?

Yes 1

No 2

IF "Yes" RECORD DETAILS BELOW

Height of mother (without shoes)_____cms.
                 (to nearest whole number)

14 Would you be willing to find out your husband's height for when I call the next time? (ASK HER TO MARK IT ON A WALL OR DOOR FOR YOU TO MEASURE)

Yes 1

No 2

IF "Yes" RECORD DETAILS DURING FINAL INTERVIEW

Height of father_____cms. (to nearest whole number)

With shoes   1
Without shoes 2

IF MOTHER KNOWS HEIGHT OF HUSBAND WITHOUT MEASURING IT:

Height of father_____ft._____ins. (to nearest inch)

With shoes   1
Without shoes 2

15 Have there been any of the following circumstances present **during the time you have been keeping the record book** which might have affected your child's usual pattern of feeding?

		Yes	No
(a)	Child has been teething	1	2
(b)	Child has been unwell	1	2
(c)	Some other member of the family has been ill	1	2
(d)	Your husband has not been working (e.g. on holiday)	1	2
(e)	You have been entertaining visitors	1	2
(f)	Have there been any other circumstances? (IF "Yes" STATE)	1	2

16 (a) Some mothers believe it is a good thing to give their children a dummy or infant feeder sometimes, while other mothers are against it. Do you think it is a good thing to give children a dummy or infant feeder sometimes?

Yes 1

No 2

(b) Have you ever given...........................(sample child) a dummy or an infant feeder?

Yes 1

No 2

IF "No" GO TO Q.17.

IF "Yes",

(c) Do you still give...........................(sample child) a dummy or infant feeder?

Yes 1

No 2

IF "Yes" GO TO Q.16(e).

IF "No",

(d) At what age did he/she stop using it?

_____years _____months

(e) Has your child ever used a dummy or infant feeder just on its own, without anything on/in it? (RECORD BELOW). Has your child ever used a dummy or infant feeder with water only? (REPEAT FOR OTHERS BELOW)

	Yes	No
On its own	1	2
Water only	1	2
Milk only	1	2
Sugar	1	2
Syrup, jam or honey	1	2
SHOW CARD Any of these vitamin supplements	1	2
Anything else? (STATE)	1	2

OFFICE USE ONLY

42

43

44

45

46

103

17   (a)   Have you a refrigerator or the use of one?

Yes	1
No	2

IF "No" GO TO Q.17(c).
IF "Yes",

(b)   Do you use it for storing milk?

Yes	1
No	2

ASK ALL

(c)   Does............(sample child) like drinking milk?

Yes	1
No	2

(d)   Do you get welfare milk tokens for free or reduced milk for:

	Yes	No
(i) Yourself?	1	2
(ii) ....(sample child)?	1	2
(iii) Any other children?	1	2

IF NO CHILDREN GET WELFARE MILK GO TO Q.18, OTHERWISE:

(e)   How many other children do you have welfare milk
tokens for?   (STATE NO.)   _____

(f)   Are any of the children who you get welfare milk tokens
for under one year old?

Yes	1
No	2

IF "Yes"

(g)   Is the milk for this child (these children) National
Dried Milk or bottled milk?

National Dried	1
Bottled	2

**COMPLETE THE FOLLOWING SECTION ONLY IF THE SAMPLE CHILD
IS 1½ YEARS OR MORE OLD**

18   (a)   It would be helpful if your child were to have his/her teeth looked at by a dentist
as this would tell us more about the effects of what children eat. This would
not, of course, involve any treatment. Would you be willing to take him/her to see
a dentist at the local clinic on a convenient day?

Yes	1
No	2.

IF "Yes" EXPLAIN ARRANGEMENTS AND ASK:

(b)   It is possible that a medical examination can be arranged at the same time
If so, would you be willing to have him/her examined?

Yes	1
No	2

**NOW CHECK ENTRIES IN THE DIARY, COMPLETE STAT NS/13 APPENDIX
AND COLLECT INFORMATION ABOUT FATHER'S HEIGHT (Page 8).**

IF MOTHER HAS BEEN SELECTED FOR REPEAT SURVEY: Ask if she would
agree to keep another week's record.

Agreed	1
Did not agree	2

If she agrees, leave new record book completed with name, address, etc., and
arrange to collect it. When collecting it, repeat all checking action.

Interviewer's signature ....

Date...

B2-Nutrition Survey (Young Children)

DIETARY RECORD BOOK

STAT NS/13
JN.46156

Name of child _____

Name of mother _____

Address _____

_____

_____

APPOINTMENTS

DAY	DATE	TIME

Any information you give will be used for statistical purposes and your name and address is known only to the British Market Research Bureau, the Government Social Survey and the Ministry of Health (or the Health Departments for Scotland and Wales), who will use it only in connection with the present survey or in any inquiry of a medical, dental or nutritional nature following on this one. Your identity will not be revealed outside the organisations just mentioned or in any publication of the results of this survey.

USING THE RECORD BOOK

SOME GENERAL POINTS

On the next page are some general points which will help you in filling in the record book
If you have any problems please ask the interviewer

105

- Write down **EVERYTHING** your child has to eat or drink (NOT ONLY the food and drink taken at main meals). Include any tonics, vitamin preparations, or medicines that your child may take.
- Begin a **NEW** double page for each day. If necessary, more than one double page can be used for one day's record.
- Write in the day of the week and the date at the top of each page.
- Write in, in COLUMN 1, the time at which the meal, snack or item of food or drink was eaten or drunk.
- Write descriptions of the food or drink in COLUMN 2 and enter their weights in COLUMNS 3 and 4, using a new line for each item of food or drink.
- Fill in **every day,** in the space provided at the bottom of the right hand page, the amount of milk you **bought** that day and the time your child went to bed at night.

HOW TO DESCRIBE THE FOOD AND DRINK

It is very important to us that you describe in detail everything your child eats and drinks and whether it is **cooked** or **not.** Here are a few examples to help you:

LIKE THIS	NOT	LIKE THIS
Cod fried in batter	NOT	Fish
Lamb chop, lean and fat	NOT	Lamb
Boiled cabbage	NOT	Vegetables
Tinned rice pudding	NOT	Rice pudding
Smarties	NOT	Sweets
Stewed apple	NOT	Apple
Fried tomato	NOT	Tomato
Wholemeal brown bread	NOT	Bread

If something is made up of several things, like a sandwich or a cup of coffee, record each part on a separate line. Here are two examples:

LIKE THIS	NOT	LIKE THIS
Bread Margarine Cheese	NOT	Sandwich
Coffee powder Water Milk Sugar	NOT	Cup of coffee

HOW TO WEIGH THE FOOD AND DRINK

- All the food and drink must be weighed on the scales we have left you when it is served.
- The big numbers on the scale are ounces and the little numbers between them are one-sixth ounces. First write in the big numbers in COLUMN 3 and then write in the small number in COLUMN 4. If the item weighs less than one ounce, write in "O" in COLUMN 3.

Some items (e.g. an apple, a biscuit, a slice of bread) can be weighed directly on the scale. Write things like this in as follows:—

Time Served	Description of food or drink Use one line or more for each item	Weight served oz	Weight served $\frac{1}{4}$ oz	Weight left over oz	Weight left over $\frac{1}{4}$ oz	Please tick items left over
(1)	(2)	(3)	(4)	(5)	(6)	(7)
11.00 am	Raw Apple	3	4	0	5	√ Core

● Other things can only be weighed on a plate or in a cup or glass. For these things first of all weigh the plate (or cup, or glass). Then put the first thing on the plate, e.g. mashed potato, and weigh the plate together with the mashed potato; then put the next thing on the plate, e.g. tinned runner beans, and weigh the plate with the mashed potato, and the tinned runner beans; go on in this way until everything is on the plate. Here is an example of how to write all this in the diary:—

Time Served	Description of food or drink Use one line or more for each item	Weight served oz	Weight served $\frac{1}{4}$ oz	Weight left over oz	Weight left over $\frac{1}{4}$ oz	Please tick items left over
(1)	(2)	(3)	(4)	(5)	(6)	(7)
12.15 pm	Plate	4	2	4	5	
	Mashed potato with milk	5	1			
	Tinned runner beans	5	5			√
	Stewed hare	7	3			
	Gravy	8	0			

Here is another example about a cup of tea:—

10.00 am	Cup	3	4	None		
	Milk	4	2			
	Sugar	4	5			
	Tea	7	3			

FOOD LEFT OVER

You will see from the examples above that we want you to weigh and write in everything that is left over. This includes things like bones, egg-shells and apple-cores as well as things one can eat. COLUMNS 5, 6 and 7 are to be used for left-overs. The points below will show you how to weigh and write in the left-overs.

● If anything at all is left over on a plate (or in a cup), weigh the plate (or the cup) with the things left over on it, and write in the weight in COLUMNS 5 and 6 on the same line on which you wrote the "plate" when you first weighed it empty.

● If nothing is left over, write in "NONE" (see the example about the cup of tea).

- Put a tick in COLUMN 7 on the same line as the item of food that is left over. You will see in the example above that some runner beans have been left over. If more than one thing has been left over you will put more than one tick, e.g. if in the example above some mashed potatoes had been left over then you would also put a tick in COLUMN 7 on the same line as mashed potato.

- If what is left over is something you cannot eat (e.g. bones, shell, core), as well as making a tick **WRITE IN** what is left over in COLUMN 7. In the above example you may write in "Bone" on the same line as Stewed Hare.

- If something is spilt, write in about how much of the food (or drink) served you think was spilt, e.g. "About ¼ spilt".

- If, as in the example above of the apple, something is weighed without a plate or a cup, then you write in the weight left over and what is left over on the same line as the food.

THINGS WHICH CANNOT BE WEIGHED

Please weigh everything you can. Some things, however, you may not be able to weigh because of their size or because they are eaten away from home. However, we still want you to write them in. Here is how:

- Sweets, chocolate, ice-cream and very small things: write in the type, size and price, and the amount or number eaten (e.g. 3d bar of milk chocolate, 7 Opal Fruits, 6d ice-cream, 2 salted peanuts, 1 vitamin B tablet).

- Items served from spoons: write down whether it is a teaspoon (and what size), dessert spoon or tablespoon, and what was in it (e.g. 1 small tablespoon of cod liver oil).

- Medicines: write down the type of medicine (if you know it, or if not what complaint it is for), how much is given, whether it is liquid or tablet, whether it is given with jam or sugar, etc. (e.g. 2 tablespoons of sweet liquid for sore throat, or 2 aspirins crushed in a teaspoon of jam).

- When your child eats away from home (in a café or with friends) write in what the child eats in the separate notebook we have given you, like this.

Eaten in
a café at
12.30 pm
{
Small dish tomato soup
1 roast potato
1 slice of lean roast beef
1 large tablespoon of peas
Gravy
Small slice of apple pie
Custard
Teaspoon of sugar (sprinkled over top of the pie)

Then when you return home copy into your record book the time at which the food was eaten in COLUMN 1, and copy the items of food or drink eaten into COLUMN 2.

Day of Week: _____

Date:. _____

PLEASE WRITE DOWN AS CLEARLY AS YOU CAN EVERYTHING
YOUR CHILD DRINKS OR EATS TODAY

Time served e.g. 5 p.m.	Description of food or drink Use one line or more per item	Weight served		Weight left over		Tick items left over	OFFICE USE ONLY													
							Cumulative dishes								Single dishes					
							R & L		Food Code	Q		U	P		Food Code	Q		U	P	
		oz	$\frac{1}{6}$ oz	oz	$\frac{1}{6}$ oz		oz	$\frac{1}{6}$		oz	$\frac{1}{6}$					oz	$\frac{1}{6}$			
(1)	(2)	(3)	(4)	(5)	(6)	(7)														

1. How much fresh milk did you **buy** altogether today? _____ pints
2. What time did your child go to bed (at night) ? _____ p.m.

109

TRIAL RECORD
TO BE COMPLETED BY THE MOTHER WITH THE INTERVIEWER

Day of Week: _____

Date: _____

PLEASE WRITE DOWN AS CLEARLY AS YOU CAN EVERYTHING YOUR CHILD EATS OR DRINKS TODAY

When served	Description of food or drink Use one line or more per item	Weight served		Weight Left Over		Tick items Left Over
		oz	$\frac{1}{8}$ oz	oz	$\frac{1}{8}$ oz	
(1)	(2)	(3)	(4)	(5)	(6)	(7)

TO BE COMPLETED BY INTERVIEWER AT END OF WEEK'S RECORD

Ascertain from participant and indicate answers to each of the following questions:

1   **Tea**   Does your child drink tea that is . . . WEAK/MEDIUM/STRONG/DOES NOT SERVE (Medium =1 spoon (or scoop) of tea, whatever size, or 1 tea bag per person plus 1 for the pot. Anything less is weak, anything more is strong.)

2   **Coffee**   Does your child have coffee that is . . . WEAK/MEDIUM/STRONG/DOES NOT SERVE. (In their own opinion).

3   **Porridge**   Does your child have porridge that is made with . . . ALL WATER/ WATERED MILK/ALL MILK/DOES NOT SERVE.

4   **Soup**   Does your child have soup that is made with . . . ALL WATER/WATERED MILK/ALL MILK/NOTHING ADDED/DOES NOT SERVE.

5   **Milk**   If the sample child drank fresh milk during the last week was it . . . JERSEY/ ORDINARY.

If the sample child drank dried milk during the last week was it described in the record book as . . . DRY WEIGHT PLUS WATER/MADE UP WEIGHT.

IF "MADE UP WEIGHT"
How many ounces of powder were used to how many ounces of water

_____Powder

_____ Water

6   **Bread**   If there are any unweighed bread entries, please weigh a typical slice_____oz. _____1/6 oz.

7   **Meat**   Is the meat eaten by the sample child usually . . . LEAN/LEAN AND FAT.

8   **Teaspoonsful**   If any items served have been recorded as teaspoonsful (and no weight given), is the teaspoon usually used . . . SMALL/MEDIUM/LARGE and is it used . . . HEAPED/NOT HEAPED.

Have you checked through the record book to ensure that the following are properly recorded?

	Check completed (initial)
1 **Bread and butter sandwiches:** Col. 2 Cols. 3 and 4 Bread Weight of bread Butter Weight of bread and butter Filling Weight of bread and butter and filling	
2 **Orange juice:** to be noted if fresh, tinned (with or without sugar), squash or "welfare".	
3 **Cod liver oil:** to be noted if "welfare".	
4 **Milk:** to be noted if condensed, evaporated, dried. If dried, to be noted whether National Dried or brand name given and whether full cream or half cream.	
5 **Bread and toast:** to be noted if Hovis, Wholemeal, brown, white, starch reduced, crispbread, etc.	
6 **Stews:** contents to be described e.g. beef, carrots, onions, thick gravy.	

B3-Nutrition Survey of Pre-School Children

MEDICAL EXAMINATION

	For office use

A. Name of child ....

   Address ....

   ....

   ....

   Date of birth ....

   Sex ....

B. Local authority ....

   Date and time of dental examination ....

   Address where examination
      will take place ....

   Arrangements for medical
      examination made by Med. 2..

C. **Details of examination**

   **Where alternative answers are given, delete those which
   are inapplicable.** Any necessary comments and elaborations
   should be entered where indicated.

1 **Hospital**   Has the child been in hospital in the last six months?
             No
             Yes—give reasons ....

             ....

             ....

2 **Illness**   Is the child ill, i.e. at the time of examination?
             No
             Yes—give details ....

             ....

             ....

3 **Obesity**   Obese
             Plump
             Normal
             Thin
             Very thin

4 **Posture**   Normal
   (standing)   Lordosis
             Kyphosis
             Scoliosis
             Other

/5.

5 **Physique**   Satisfactory
   (physical   Unsatisfactory—give details..
   condition)

   ....

   ....

6 **Gums** (i)   Bases of upper incisors bleed after
                   manual pressure   No/Yes
        (ii)   Gingivitis (not localised to one
                   tooth) present   No/Yes..............................

   ....

   ....

7 **Lips**   Angular stomatitis   No
                                      Yes ....

   ....

8 **Tongue**   Normal
                Abnormal—specify ....

   ....

9 **Scurvy**   No
                Yes—Major bruises
                     Petechial haemorrhages
                     Bleeding gums
                     X-ray
                     Other

   ....

   ....

10 **Rickets**   No
                  Yes—Active
                       Healed
                       Radiologically confirmed No/Yes

11 **Other information relevant to nutrition**

Signature of doctor ....

Date of examination..

B4-Nutrition Survey
of Pre-School Children

DENTAL EXAMINATION   STAT/NS 8

Date of examination ....

Name of mother...

Name of child   ....

Address ....

....

Date of birth ....

1   Please record the condition of the teeth on the chart below, **according to the instructions overleaf.**

| E | D | C | B | A | A | B | C | D | E |

2   Please complete the "score" of the above record as follows:—

	Incisors		**Other teeth**	
Number of teeth—				
(i) sound (including erupting teeth)	....		....	
(ii) unerupted	....		....	
(iii) missing because of trauma*	....		....	
(iv) filled	....	**Total def†**	....	**Total def†**
(v) carious but not filled	....	....	....	....
(vi) extracted because of caries or sepsis, etc*	....		....	

*Teeth known to have been lost from injury or accident should be included at (iii); all other missing teeth should be included at (vi).

†i.e. items (iv), (v) and (vi).

....
Signature of examining dental officer

114

Instructions for completion of dental chart

The symbols and a specimen completed chart for recording the condition and history of the teeth are shown below. A tooth is counted as erupted (i.e present and sound) if any part of it can be touched by a probe.

Symbols

Tooth present and sound	\	at left hand bottom of square
Tooth unerupted	U	
Tooth extracted because of caries or sepsis etc.	X	
Tooth missing because of trauma	—	
Root present	+	
Cavity present	O	} According to outline
Filling present	●	}
Tooth erupting	E	

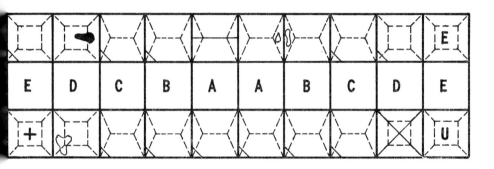

This survey is not concerned with the amount of dental treatment required, but with life caries experience, which is the actual experience—past, shown as teeth which have been filled or extracted, and present, shown as carious cavities.

The examination should be made by good natural daylight or artificial light—radiographs are not recommended. Plane mouth mirrors and sharp probes should be used and, to ensure that the probes are uniformly effective, each one should be used for no more than 8 children.

In assessing active caries, no abnormality should be reported as carious unless there is an actual break of surface continuity in which the probe penetrates to the dentine. In recording a cavity, the surfaces actually involved should be shown. A cavity in a proximal surface is a one-surface lesion if the occlusal surface is intact, even though its restoration will eventually involve the occlusal surface.

15. Appendix C
Apparatus for anthropometry

(1) Introduction

One of the limiting factors in a survey which involves domiciliary visits is the weight and portability of the apparatus. A further consideration, relating to the anthropometry of random samples of children to whom the interviewer is a stranger, is that the machines for weighing and measuring must not be alarming in character. These two considerations governed the design of the apparatus used in the survey. The apparatus described below met these requirements. Tables A39 and 40 (p 66) show that the standard deviations of the mean height and weight measurements in the present study tend to be slightly larger than the standard deviations in other studies made in 8 different countries reported by Heimendinger (1964), which suggests that our apparatus was less accurate. But it needs to be remembered that the measurements were made by 12 different observers, each measuring only about 3 subjects per week in a study that lasted for a year. Further, the measurements were made under the varying conditions of many different homes. Though we have not the details of all the other studies these disadvantages may not have operated in them. As epidemiological tools for the purposes of the present study the pieces of apparatus described below proved effective as well as being practicable.

(2) Weight

It was decided to produce something which the child would identify as a swing and therefore associate with pleasure (*Frontispiece I*). The apparatus consisted of three main parts: (A) a horizontal arm, to which a spring dial weighing machine was hooked and from which a seat was suspended by ropes. The arm was designed to slot into the top of a standard door. Rubber gaitering protected the paint and in practice there were no complaints that the door was in any way damaged. (B) the swing seat was suspended from ropes which also passed through the ends of horizontal wooden bars so as to form a cage at the sides and back. (C) in the front a bar was fitted which would be raised and lowered in the rope so as to prevent the child from falling out.

Clothing was weighed separately on the scales used for dietary recording and the appropriate deduction made.

(3) Height

It was necessary to measure both the parents in the standing position and the child supine. Again the apparatus was in three parts (*Frontispiece II*): a stainless steel platform (A) with an angled plane and with slots cut so as to contain a grip in the zero end of an ordinary steel tape (B). To the cowling of the steel tape there was attached (C), a flat flange which could be applied to the top of the child's (or parents') head in a plane at right angles to the long axis of the extended tape. There is here a potential error because the rectiliniarity of the tape to both the footpiece and the headpiece had to be judged by eye. Trials were made using 2 tapes, one on each side of the child's body, but the difficulties of their use were greater than appeared to be warranted by any increase in accuracy (and in practice the standard errors of the means of the measurements justified this decision). When measuring children, the footpiece was placed against a wall adjoining a smooth (i.e. non-carpeted) floor. The child lay on his back, his head held as specified in the IBP handbook (Weiner and Lourie 1969). The tape, inserted into the slot, was extended, and the headpiece appropriately used. The interviewers were instructed that it was better to have no measurement at all rather than one which was suspect because the child was fractious or for any reason could not be persuaded into the right position. The parents were measured standing on the footpiece, with the tape stretched vertically against a smooth wall (i.e. one without skirting) or other surface such as a door. The head was extended and held in the position specified (IBP handbook) with one hand, the headpiece being applied with the other. In some cases where the interviewer did not meet the father his reported height was used.

16. Appendix D
Medical Examinations

(1) Table A2 (p 38) shows that the children who were medically examined were fairly evenly represented in the three family size groups of the three older age groups.

(2) Table A41 (p 67), which includes all four age groups, compares the mean daily intakes of energy and nutrients of the children who were examined with those of the children who were not, and shows that for most nutrients there was no significant difference between the two groups. The intake of vitamin D of children medically examined was significantly lower and that of pyridoxine and the percentage of energy from protein significantly higher, than that of children not medically examined, but there seems to be no obvious reason for these differences. Thus, although only a small group of children was examined the group was similar in nutrient intake to the survey group as a whole. Table A41 also shows that the mean intakes of most nutrients by the much larger number of children who were medically examined in the pilot survey in 1963 (Ministry of Health, 1968) were not appreciably different from the intakes by those who were, and were not, medically examined in 1967–68. The exceptions were the intakes of nicotinic acid and vitamin C which were substantially greater in 1967–68, and vitamin D intake which was less. The consumption of "added sugars" and, to a lesser extent, the total intake of carbohydrate, had also risen.

(3) The physical condition of all 95 children who were examined in this survey was described as satisfactory. None was said to be obese, and only one child was recorded as thin. None of the children had angular stomatitis, haemorrhages in the skin or any abnormalities indicative of rickets or of any other vitamin deficiency.

17. Appendix E
Dental Health

The dental health of the pre-school child as judged by the results of the Nutrition Survey 1967-68

J Rodgers
Senior Dental Officer, DHSS

(1) The Sample

(a) The parents of all survey children in the age groups $1\frac{1}{2}$–$2\frac{1}{2}$, $2\frac{1}{2}$–$3\frac{1}{2}$ and $3\frac{1}{2}$–$4\frac{1}{2}$ years were invited to take them for dental examination and 66% of the children for whom a dietary record was obtained were examined. The percentages of children examined in the different age/family size groups are shown in Table E1.

Table E1 : *Percentage of children who were dentally examined in the different age groups and different family sizes*

Age group (years)	Number of children in family under 15 years of age		
	1 or 2	3	4 or more
$1\frac{1}{2}$–$2\frac{1}{2}$	71	70	63
$2\frac{1}{2}$–$3\frac{1}{2}$	66	63	61
$3\frac{1}{2}$–$4\frac{1}{2}$	67	69	59

(b) A slightly higher percentage of younger children from smaller families was examined. Social factors influenced whether or not children were brought for examination since social classes IV and V had the lowest response rate (Table E2), but response was not related to the age at which the mother left school.

Table E2: *Number of children of different social classes who were dentally examined*

Social class	Number eligible for examination	Percentage of eligible children examined
I and II	201	67
III Non-Manual	97	82
III Manual	544	66
IV and V	246	60

(c) There was a gap in time between home interview and dental examination, and mothers who co-operated willingly with interviewers may have lost enthusiasm due to this. A second appointment was offered to mothers who failed to keep the first.

(2) Dental examination

The examination was made by local authority dental officers and the technique was standardized so as to minimize inter-observer error as far as possible. The examinations were carried out in good light. All probes were discarded after being used for 8 examinations. The examining officers were instructed to record caries only where there was a break in the surface continuity of the enamel through which the probe penetrated to the dentine. The total numbers of decayed, extracted and filled teeth (def) and the def for incisor teeth only were recorded separately.

(3) Results of the clinical examination

(a) Table E3 shows that in all age groups the mean def both for all teeth and for incisors was usually greatest in children from large families.

Table E3: *The number of decayed, extracted and filled teeth in children of different ages from families of different size*[1]

Age group (years)	Number of children in family	Number of children examined	Number of teeth	
			Mean total def	Mean incisor def
$1\frac{1}{2}$–$2\frac{1}{2}$	1 or 2	110	0.2	0.1
	3	94	0.4	0.1
	4 or more	66	0.5	0.2
$2\frac{1}{2}$–$3\frac{1}{2}$	1 or 2	97	1.7	0.3
	3	92	1.7	0.4
	4 or more	70	1.8	0.4
$3\frac{1}{2}$–$4\frac{1}{2}$	1 or 2	74	2.9	0.3
	3	82	2.8	0.5
	4 or more	53	3.4	0.9

[1] Children under 15 years of age.

(b) The dental health of the children in most age and family size groups was better in families of social classes I and II (Table E5).

(c) As a basis for comparing mean intakes by gradations of dental health, children were classified according to the total numbers of def teeth, with the results shown in Table E4.

Table E4: *The distribution of children of different ages in each of the def groups indicating a gradation in dental health*

Total number of def teeth	Age group (years)					
	$1\frac{1}{2}$–$2\frac{1}{2}$		$2\frac{1}{2}$–$3\frac{1}{2}$		$3\frac{1}{2}$–$4\frac{1}{2}$	
	Number	% of those examined	Number	% of those examined	Number	% of those examined
None	229	85	145	56	84	40
1–4	35	13	76	29	63	30
5–8	6	2	27	11	43	21
9 or more	0	0	11	4	19	9
not examined	124	—	148	—	110	—

(d) Table E6 shows the mean daily intakes of energy and certain nutrients in each of these groups. There was some indication of an increase in the number of def teeth with an increased intake of "added sugars". Higher def rates were associated with lower intakes of calcium and milk. Intakes of vitamins A, D and C were also less in those

119

Table E5: *The number of decayed, extracted and filled teeth of children from families of different sizes[1] and different social classes*

Age group (years)	Number of children in family	Social class							
		I and II		III Non-Manual		III Manual		IV and V	
		all teeth def	incisors def	all teeth def	incisors def	all teeth def	incisors def	all teeth def	incisors def
$1\frac{1}{2}-2\frac{1}{2}$	1 or 2	0.2	0.0	0.6	0.3	0.2	0.1	0.2	0.1
	3	0.1	0.0	1.3	0.4	0.3	0.2	0.6	0.0
	4 or more	0.8	0.2	1.0	1.0	0.3	0.1	0.7	0.3
$2\frac{1}{2}-3\frac{1}{2}$	1 or 2	1.7	0.1	0.9	0.0	2.2	0.6	1.4	0.1
	3	1.1	0.4	1.5	0.2	2.0	0.5	1.7	0.5
	4 or more	1.2	0.2	2.2	0.0	1.5	0.4	3.1	0.9
$3\frac{1}{2}-4\frac{1}{2}$	1 or 2	1.5	0.0	2.4	0.2	3.3	0.5	4.2	0.4
	3	2.5	0.3	3.4	1.0	2.6	0.7	3.6	0.6
	4 or more	2.0	0.3	4.7	2.0	4.2	1.2	2.4	0.4

[1]Children under 15 years of age

children with a higher def rate. Apparent inconsistencies in the findings could have been due to small numbers in some groupings.

(e) It is interesting that the third of the children producing diet records who were not dentally examined had in many age groups higher intakes of energy and nutrients. It could be that poor dental health was an important factor in the mother's decision to allow a dental examination or there may be some other social or economic factor which cannot be deduced from the results of this survey.

(f) The use of a dummy or reservoir feeder was related to social class—72% of mothers in social classes I, II and III Non-Manual, compared with 55% in social classes III Manual, IV and V said their children had never used one. This difference did not seem to be associated with family size. It is not unlikely that some under-recording occurs when a question such as this is asked, particularly of mothers in the higher social classes, but the fact that the interviewers were not nurses and would not in any sense be critical may have encouraged truthful answers. Dummies were often dipped in sugar and syrups and the use of a dipped dummy was included with the use of a reservoir feeder. Reservoir feeders consist of a small glass container with a rubber teat and they usually contain a vitamin syrup or sweetened water or other liquid. The non-nutritive use of a dummy or feeder was recorded under "on own or with water only". The children whose parents stated that they had never used a dummy or reservoir feeder were generally in better dental health than the others. In the age group $3\frac{1}{2}$–$4\frac{1}{2}$ years, $7\frac{1}{2}$% of children were still using reservoir feeders or dummies. In the age group $1\frac{1}{2}$–$2\frac{1}{2}$ years, both the mean total def and incisor def were larger in the children who used a reservoir container filled with sweetened syrupy fluids than in those who did not use the feeder, or those in which the container was only filled with water. In the older age groups the evidence that there is a relationship between caries and the use of sweetened syrupy fluids in reservoir feeders is less conclusive (Table E7).

(g) In family size 3, there were 9 children aged $1\frac{1}{2}$–$2\frac{1}{2}$ years who were described as having used a feeder with additives but who had discontinued the practice for over 6 months prior to the week of the survey. These 9 children had a mean total def of 0·7 but no incisor caries. There were 11 children aged $2\frac{1}{2}$–$3\frac{1}{2}$ years from families with 1 or 2 children who had discontinued using a reservoir feeder with additives more than 6 months previously; the mean total def of these children was 3·2, and of the incisor def 1·0. These findings, though they appear contradictory, are less surprising when one considers that the latter group had been using a reservoir feeder with additives for one year longer than the former.

(h) Since older children used dummies and reservoir feeders less frequently, the average def totals for all teeth and for incisor teeth were compared in children who had ceased to use the feeder for more than 6 months with those who had never used it (Table E8).

(i) The questionnaire noted the timing of the last meal, i.e. whether it occurred within $\frac{1}{4}$ of an hour or less of bedtime, or more than $\frac{1}{4}$ hour but less than $\frac{1}{2}$ hour, or more than $\frac{1}{2}$ hour but less than 1 hour before; or whether it was irregular or not stated. No attempt was made to classify the meal itself as to its cariogenicity although its content would be noted in the dietary records. No conclusions could be drawn from the statistical recording of these facts and their relation to the number of def teeth. There are many small children who have an afternoon nap and it is not unlikely that they have a snack beforehand which may make the timing of the last meal and its relationship to bedtime less meaningful.

(j) The range of bedtimes is shown in Table E9. It is perhaps surprising that 3% of the survey children were said usually to go to bed after 10 p.m.

(k) The use of wholemeal bread was noted in order to assess whether or not such bread had a protective factor for children's teeth. In this survey, few of the children ate wholemeal bread and there was no relationship between the number of def teeth and the consumption of wholemeal bread.

121

Table E6: *Mean daily intake and intake/1000 kcal of energy, some nutrients and milk, for groups of children of different ages classified according to the number of def teeth*

Number of def teeth	Age group (years)					
	$1\frac{1}{2}$–$2\frac{1}{2}$		$2\frac{1}{2}$–$3\frac{1}{2}$		$3\frac{1}{2}$–$4\frac{1}{2}$	
	Mean daily intake	Intake per 1000 kcal	Mean daily intake	Intake per 1000 kcal	Mean daily intake	Intake per 1000 kcal
Energy						
kcal None	1261	—	1358	—	1484	—
MJ	5.3		5.7		6.2	
1–4	1246	—	1460	—	1372	—
	5.2		6.1		5.7	
5–8	1191	—	1462	—	1441	—
	5.0		6.1		6.0	
9 or more	—	—	1284	—	1398	—
			5.4		5.9	
Not examined	1270	—	1410	—	1535	—
	5.3		5.9		6.4	
Carbohydrate						
g None	164	130	178	131	197	134
1–4	166	133	194	133	186	136
5–8	163	137	193	132	195	135
9 or more	—	—	168	132	186	134
Not examined	164	130	189	134	207	136
"Added sugars"[1]						
g None	56.7	45.0	62.2	45.7	67.9	46.5
1–4	61.1	48.9	64.8	45.0	67.3	49.3
5–8	58.8	49.1	72.6	50.2	73.7	50.8
9 or more	—	—	58.0	46.0	67.3	49.4
Not examined	55.6	44.3	66.3	47.3	70.3	46.6
Calcium						
mg None	690	560	660	490	690	460
1–4	640	520	690	480	630	460
5–8	560	470	660	450	650	460
9 or more	—	—	580	460	610	440
Not examined	720	580	650	460	670	440
Vitamin A						
iu None	2540	2010	2300	1680	2700	1840
µg	760	600	690	500	810	550
1–4	2420	1910	2490	1670	2350	1640
	730	570	750	500	710	490
5–8	1440	1220	2260	1600	2200	1590
	430	370	680	480	660	480
9 or more	—	—	1990	1570	1700	1160
	—	—	600	470	510	350
Not examined	2520	2000	2020	1480	2380	1550
	760	600	610	440	710	470

[1]"Added sugars" are defined as any sugars added during cooking, preparation or manufacture as distinct from the naturally occurring carbohydrates of the basic foods. With a few exceptions these sugars were added in the form of sucrose. Total carbohydrate is expressed as monosaccharides and added sugars as disaccharides. Confectionery (sweets) and preserves were the foods which contributed mainly to a high intake of "added sugar".

122

Table E6 (cont.)

	Number of def teeth	Age group (years)					
		1½–2½		2½–3½		3½–4½	
		Mean daily intake	Intake per 1000 kcal	Mean daily intake	Intake per 1000 kcal	Mean daily intake	Intake per 1000 kcal
Vitamin D							
iu	None	117	94	73	53	82	56
µg		2.9	2.4	1.8	1.3	2.1	1.4
	1–4	87	73	95	64	82	55
		2.2	1.8	2.4	1.6	2.1	1.4
	5–8	47	42	79	58	71	49
		1.2	1.1	2.0	1.5	1.8	1.2
	9 or more	—	—	101	81	42	28
				2.5	2.0	1.1	0.7
	Not examined	122	97	80	58	66	45
		3.1	2.4	2.0	1.5	1.7	1.1
Vitamin C							
mg	None	42	34	37	29	47	33
	1–4	39	29	42	30	34	25
	5–8	25	21	38	27	34	24
	9 or more	—	—	29	24	26	18
	Not examined	38	32	34	25	37	25
Milk							
oz	None	13.6	—	12.5	—	12.6	—
	1–4	12.5	—	12.6	—	11.4	—
	5–8	10.1	—	11.8	—	11.7	—
	9 or more	—	—	9.8	—	10.5	—
	Not examined	14.4	—	11.7	—	12.2	—

Table E7: *The number of total and incisor def teeth in children of different ages from families of different size according to whether a dummy or reservoir feeder was used or not*

No. of children in family under 15 years	Used dummy or reservoir feeder	Age group (years)								
		$1\frac{1}{2}-2\frac{1}{2}$			$2\frac{1}{2}-3\frac{1}{2}$			$3\frac{1}{2}-4\frac{1}{2}$		
		No. of children	Total def	Incisor def	No. of children	Total def	Incisor def	No. of children	Total def	Incisor def
1 or 2	Never	69	0.1	0.0	54	1.5	0.3	39	2.8	0.2
	Alone or with water	17	0.1	0.0	7	2.1	0.3	4	3.0	0.5
	With additive[1]	11	1.3	0.7	9	3.0	0.6	1	1.0	0.0
3	Never	48	0.3	0.0	57	1.6	0.3	43	2.7	0.5
	Alone or with water	17	0.8	0.3	7	4.0	1.6	4	3.2	1.3
	With additive[1]	6	1.0	0.7	4	1.3	0.3	1	5.0	0.0
4 or more	Never	43	0.6	0.2	42	2.0	0.4	31	3.8	1.0
	Alone or with water	7	0.0	0.0	7	0.6	0.1	2	1.5	0.0
	With additive[1]	5	1.4	0.4	5	2.4	0.6	3	0.0	0.0

[1]With additive means that the reservoir feeder was filled with a sweetened fluid or syrup.

Table E8: *Comparison of mean def totals for all teeth and for incisors only in children aged $3\frac{1}{2}$–$4\frac{1}{2}$ years of different family sizes who had stopped using a feeder with additives[1] for more than 6 months and in children who had never used a feeder*

No. children in family under 15 years	Use of feeder	No. children	All teeth def	Incisors def
1–2	Never	39	2.8	0.2
	Discontinued	18	3.2	0.4
3	Never	43	2.7	0.5
	Discontinued	14	3.7	0.8
4 or more	Never	31	3.8	1.0
	Discontinued	8	2.5	0.8

[1]With additive means that the reservoir feeder was filled with a sweetened fluid or syrup.

Table E9: *The number of children in each of the four age groups analysed according to their usual bedtime*

Bedtime		All children	Age group (years)			
			$\frac{1}{2}$–$1\frac{1}{2}$	$1\frac{1}{2}$–$2\frac{1}{2}$	$2\frac{1}{2}$–$3\frac{1}{2}$	$3\frac{1}{2}$–$4\frac{1}{2}$
Before 6	pm	7	2	3	2	—
6–7	pm	262	55	83	77	47
7–8	pm	432	67	122	126	117
8–9	pm	152	13	44	46	49
9–10	pm	39	5	9	13	12
After 10	pm	39	13	14	8	4
Variable		400	50	121	137	92
All children		1331	205	396	409	321

(4) Conclusions

(a) Though the survey was not designed primarily as a dental study, basic information as to the mean def values in each age, family size and social class group was obtained and these are quoted in the tables.

(b) There was evidence that the mean def values were greater both for all teeth and for the incisors in the younger children who used dummies or feeders filled with sweet syrupy liquids. The evidence that such liquids in feeders are associated with caries was less strong among the older age groups but here we relied on the memory of the mother. There were too few children who ate wholemeal bread to give any definite evidence of a relationship with caries; if evidence had been produced we would have examined it in relation to social factors. Similarly caries was not shown to be definitely related to eating just before going to bed.

(c) There were areas where no positive conclusion could be drawn due to the number of children in the categories being small. Larger numbers of children with caries may require to be dentally examined in order that the findings be more definite. Nevertheless the survey provided an opportunity to examine dentally a representative sample of very young children, establish their dental condition and consider the various factors which could affect it.

125

Printed in England by Burrup, Mathieson & Co., Ltd., London SE1 0NX,
and published by Her Majesty's Stationery Office.

Dd 290568 K8 8/75

S882794 LE

HER MAJESTY'S STATIONERY OFFICE

Government Bookshops

49 High Holborn, London WC1V 6HB
13a Castle Street, Edinburgh EH2 3AR
41 The Hayes, Cardiff CF1 1JW
Brazennose Street, Manchester M60 8AS
Southey House, Wine Street, Bristol BS1 2BQ
258 Broad Street, Birmingham B1 2HE
80 Chichester Street, Belfast BT1 4JY

*Government Publications are also available
through booksellers*

ISBN 0 11 320603 8